SUICIDE INTERVENTION IN THE SCHOOLS

The Guilford School Practitioner Series

EDITORS

STEPHEN N. ELLIOTT, Ph.D.
University of Wisconsin—Madison

JOSEPH C. WITT, Ph.D.
Louisiana State University, Baton Rouge

SUICIDE INTERVENTION IN THE SCHOOLS

SCOTT POLAND, Ed.D.

THE GUILFORD PRESS
New York   London

© 1989 The Guilford Press
A Division of Guilford Publications, Inc.
72 Spring Street, New York, NY 10012

Printed in the United States of America

Last digit is print number: 9 8 7 6 5 4 3 2

Library of Congress Cataloging-in-Publication Data

Poland, Scott.
    Suicide intervention in the schools / Scott Poland.
        p.   cm.—(The Guilford school practitioners series)
    Bibliography: p.
    Includes index.
    ISBN 0-89862-353-7. — ISBN 0-89862-232-8 (pbk.)
        1. Suicide—United States—Prevention.   2. Students—United
    States—Suicidal behavior.   3. Personnel service in education—
    United States.   I. Title.   II. Series.
        [DNLM: 1. Crisis intervention.   2. School Health Services.
    3. Students—psychology.   4. Suicide—in adolescence.   5. Suicide—
    prevention & control.   HV 6546 P762s.]
    HV6546.P65 1989
    371.4′6—dc 19
    DNLM/DLC
    for Library of Congress   88-36988
                                                                   CIP

Preface

I will never forget some of the things that my father said to me 2 days before he shot himself. My father made a special trip to visit my brother in one state and myself in another. He said that he did not want to live to be an old man and feared that he might have to be taken care of. He also told me what personal possessions he wanted to leave me. I was worried about him, but did not grasp that he was contemplating suicide. Like most people, I was not comfortable with the topic and did not respond in a direct, caring manner. My father said his farewell to me, went home, and shot himself the day after his 53rd birthday.

As this description indicates, my father's words and actions gave very definite clues that he was planning to commit suicide, but I did not detect these. I had not received any formal training in suicide prevention, despite the fact that I was a graduate student in psychology. This is the case for most of our population, despite the fact that suicide is the seventh leading cause of death across all age groups and the second leading cause of death among teenagers. I have also learned that previous attempts are a significant predictor of subsequent attempts. I now realize that the time that my father's gun went off, blowing a hole in the ceiling when I was 12, may not have been an accident.

I began working as a school psychologist 7 years ago and was ill prepared to deal with suicidal students. I had received no training, and there were no procedures to guide me. A call from a school nurse at a junior high school brought me into contact with a suicidal student for the first time. I will never forget the uncertainty and the fear that I felt. I wanted desperately to help, but I was unsure of how to do so, and I did not know what the role of the school should be. I have learned a lot in the last 7 years about working with suicide in the schools, and this book is written in the hope that other educators will be better prepared than I was to deal with that first suicidal student. It is a necessity in education today that we be prepared to deal with this topic.

This book contains many practical examples of how a school system can approach the topic of suicide intervention in the schools. The case examples I give are composites of suicidal students with whom I have worked. I thank the administration of the Cypress–Fairbanks (Texas) Independent School District for its support. The administration has demonstrated a great deal of confidence in the psychological staff.

The space limitations of this book do not allow for the inclusion of many supplemental materials related to procedures and other topics. For these materials, please contact me at 12318 Amado, Houston, TX 77065, or phone (713) 897-4170. Workshop presentations are also available.

Scott Poland

Contents

1

Introduction

Teenage suicide is a societal problem with tremendous implications for the schools. The schools have been reluctant even to recognize this problem, much less to devote resources toward the development of formalized prevention procedures. Harris and Crawford (1987) have commented that "unless a school has already experienced an individual or a cluster suicide, virtually no preparation appears to exist, no procedures stand ready to be put into effect, and a number of myths appear to continue to be perpetuated regarding the etiology and the warning signs of suicide" (p. vi).

At present, most suicide intervention programs in the schools are developed in the aftermath of a crisis, and there is a tendency to allow such programs to remain dormant much of the time. Much has been said about the reluctance of school administrators to work on this problem. Lennox (1987) concluded after surveying 71 suicidology professionals that a major issue is to get school administrators to agree that a program is needed. The problem is not a new one: An outbreak of suicide in European schools in the early 1900s emphasized the responsibility of the schools. Stekel, a social scientist of that period (quoted in Peck, Farberow, & Litman, 1985), commented, "[T]he school is not responsible for the suicide of its pupils, but it also does not prevent these suicides. This is its only, but perhaps its greatest, sin" (p. 158).

When a suicide does occur, there is an immediate linkage to the school, and the news media often directly report the name of the school in stories and headlines. Ross (1985a) states that it is fear and not lack of concern that results in educators' reluctance to address this problem. I have been asked by administrators, "Will we make this problem worse instead of better by attempting to work on it?" Administrators often view suicide as a problem that happens elsewhere. They also have concerns about legal

1

and liability issues. I feel very strongly that we need to address the problem openly and honestly.

Much has been written in recent years about the dramatically increased incidence of teenage suicide in the last two decades. Leder (1987) states that suicide is now the second leading cause of death among teenagers and that its incidence has tripled since 1955. Smith and Crawford (1986) estimate that from 1.5 to 2.4 million high school students have made suicide attempts. This figure is supported by Dodie Livingston, Commissioner for Children, Youth, & Families of the U.S. Department of Health and Human Services, who convened a National Conference on Youth Suicide in 1985. It is almost impossible to get exact figures on the incidence of teenage suicide, and it is a certainty that it is underreported. There is no question that suicidal students are in attendance in every secondary school in this country. The question we face is thus "What can the schools do to help?"

Much has also been written in the last several years about the causes of teenage suicide, and, in particular, the causes of the recent dramatic increase. The number of factors involved may total as many as 15, according to Leder (1987). A national survey of 11,000 teenagers themselves cited hopeless feelings and the stress of home and school; of this sample, 18% of the girls and 11% of the boys reported a prior suicide attempt (Hellmich, 1988). Emphasis has also been placed on the increased stress created by such facts of modern life as family constellation changes and substance abuse. Each individual young person has a unique set of problems, but there are common pathogens that can be identified to help us with preventive efforts. A number of warning signs have been identified and can be taught to the school community, including all who attend and work in the schools.

It is also important to pay attention to the content of student themes, poems, and artwork. This poem, written by a suicidal adolescent, gives insight into the forces and factors of teenage suicide.

A Small Flower

Come and touch me,
Smell me,
Hold me.
Please don't leave me
Out in the fields alone.
Notice me.
And use me
For a gift to someone,
For an arrangement in the den,

For anything,
But please don't toss me out
While I'm fresh.
If my leaves do turn brown
And crinkle,
Remember what I was
Before I faded away.

The topic of suicide is one that has long fascinated teenagers and one that has been prevalent in the literature for a long time. For generations, high school students have read Shakespeare's *Romeo and Juliet*, which depicts young lovers who see no alternative but suicide. More recently, the lyrics of a number of rock songs have had suicide as a theme. Elton John and Bernie Taupin wrote a song in 1972 entitled "I Think I'm Gonna Kill Myself," which graphically describes the impact that a contemplated suicide might have on society. A song entitled "Suicide Solution," written by Ozzy Osbourne, was the subject of a recent court case because the parents of a boy who committed suicide while listening to the song sued Osbourne (Coleman, 1987b).

It is not unusual for young people to ask questions about suicide and to seek out information on the subject. I have talked with parents who have been quite alarmed that their child has chosen to write a paper on suicide. Ross (1985a), commenting on the importance of providing teenagers with accurate information, states that "they want desperately to know about suicide because they are terribly attracted and terribly repelled by the idea of it" (p. 147).

There is debate about how much information a young person should be provided about suicide. Ross (1985a), in emphasizing the importance of teaching youngsters the facts about life and death, comments that suicide has intruded on the lives of most teenagers today: They may have experienced personal thoughts of suicide, they may know someone who has attempted suicide, and almost certainly they have had media exposure to the suicide of a young person. A national survey of high achievers in 1986 revealed that 46% knew a young person who had tried to commit suicide or had committed suicide, and 31% had thought about suicide themselves (Lindegard, 1986). A similar survey of high-achieving students in 1987 came up with similar figures: 45% said they knew of a teenager who had attempted suicide and 30% had considered it themselves (Hidlay, 1988). These teenagers emphasized the need for educational programs and counseling in the schools.

A consensus exists among professionals that the problem needs to be addressed through the curriculum, but professionals differ on the amount of emphasis they recommend should be placed directly on the topic of suicide. It appears clear that most teenagers turn to their friends first for help. Ross (1985a) surveyed a group of teenagers 91% of whom indicated that they would first tell a friend of their suicidal thoughts. However, teenagers often delay in seeking help for a suicidal friend.

Is it better to do nothing, and just carry on and ignore the circumstances of a suicidal death? The possibility of a contagion effect is very real, and numerous communities have had to deal with contagion. School administrators must set a course of action and be prepared to deal with the news media. The media can have tremendous influence on how the school is perceived and on the reaction of students. Schools must be prepared to deal with postvention. The suicide of a student causes much anxiety and soul-searching.

Crabb (1982) has stressed that administrators will want to get back to normal quickly, and those in counseling positions will need to advocate providing discussion for the range of emotions that students will have. Spoonhour (1985) has emphasized that parents are frightened in the aftermath of a suicide. I have worked with parents who are very concerned about their children and want to know how they can help them cope with suddenly being the survivors of a suicide. There is documentation that the survivors of suicide are now more at risk themselves (Lamb & Dunne-Maxim, 1987).

Much misinformation exists about suicide. This book contains a chapter on frequently asked questions about suicide and their answers (see Chapter 11). I have conducted in-service training sessions on suicide in several states, and have been asked many questions by school personnel at all levels and by lawmakers who are debating whether or not legislation is needed. States that have passed suicide prevention legislation include Alabama, California, Florida, New Jersey, Texas, and Wisconsin. There is growing national awareness of the need for such legislation. I helped draft the legislation in Texas and testified before the Public Education Committee of the Texas House of Representatives. In June 1987, Texas passed a resolution recommending study of the causes and factors involved in youth suicide. There has also been increased discussion of youth suicide at the national level, and several bills have been introduced before Congress. The national PTA has voiced concern over schools' reluctance to work on the problem (Kahn, 1985).

Schools need to identify resources in this area and to coordinate their own efforts with those of the appropriate community, state, and national agencies and organizations. I presented an in-service training session to all counselors, nurses, psychologists, and diagnosticians of a large school district recently, and found them to be very interested in this topic. I was surprised that no one in the large audience belonged to the American Association of Suicidology (AAS), which I perceive as an excellent resource. Chapter 12 of this book contains information about organizations, crisis centers, films, books, and curriculum guides. I hope that listing these sources will help school districts gather materials that will help them develop and implement an intervention program.

My work on this problem and on the program I have helped to develop has evolved over the years. I recommend that each school district have a crisis intervention program that is comprehensive in nature; there are many crisis situations that affect the public schools, and suicide is just one of them. Caplan (1964) has stressed that we should be involved in crisis intervention at several levels, and I have found this conceptual framework invaluable in approaching the problem of teenage suicide. Although this book only deals with suicide intervention, I advocate that schools prepare for other crisis situations as well. Many people have commented that what they learn in one crisis situation can be carried over to help them in another.

Cantor (1987) has estimated that at least 20% of teenage suicides can be prevented; Ruof and Harris (1988b) believe that as many as 80–90% of such suicides can be prevented. With a comprehensive, well-organized crisis intervention program in place, schools can do much to prevent these tragedies, and can help the school community survive if a tragedy cannot be prevented.

2

Incidence

As noted in Chapter 1, there seems to be little doubt that teenage suicide has increased dramatically in the last two decades. I have read many figures describing the incidence rate and have looked at the figures released by the Centers for Disease Control (CDC) in a 1986 report, *Youth Suicide in the United States, 1970 to 1980*.

Many writers have commented on the difficulty involved in getting accurate statistics on youth suicide. It is very common to refer to the published statistics as an underestimate. How much *has* the suicide rate risen in the last one or two decades? How should one approach school administrators and school board members with information on the incidence of youth suicide? Are there certain age, sex, or ethnic groups that are more at risk? Are there more suicides in urban areas than in rural areas? How many suicide attempts are there for each completed suicide? What do these statistics mean for the schools? These are the types of questions that I have been asked by school personnel.

The incidence of teenage suicide could be the topic of an entire book. In fact, it is often emphasized to such an extent that other aspects of the problem are neglected: I have been to in-service sessions for school personnel that focused only on incidence and not on what schools can do to work on this problem. In this chapter, I give only an overview of the topic, with an emphasis on what information is needed to convince school administrators that suicide could become a problem in their schools. My work in the schools has taught me that the incidence rate is sufficiently high that intervention programs are needed.

REPORTED CASES AND ESTIMATES
OF UNREPORTED CASES

A sampling of statistics and comments from writers on the incidence of teen suicide gives us much to think about. The Los Angeles County school system experiences approximately 300 suicides annually (Scobie, 1986). A study of New York City high school students found that 62% had thought of suicide and 9% had made an attempt (Harkavy-Friedman, Asnis, Boek, & DiFiore, 1987). Smith and Crawford (1986) studied 239 Midwestern high school students (data on 76 students from a private girls' school were excluded) and found that 62.6% had some degree of suicidal ideation, with 8.4% reporting an actual attempt. Several other studies cited by these authors found that from 10% to 15% of adolescents had made attempts. Smith and Crawford found a geographical variance of attempt rates from 8.4% of the Kansas high school students they studied to 13.0% in a California high school. They further estimated 50–120 attempts for each completed suicide, and stressed that 90% of attempters do not get medical help. They pointed out that suicide is a personal concern for one in four high school students.

The figures given above for ideation are very similar to the estimate by Ross (1985a) that 38–52% of high school students had made plans to commit suicide. We (Cohen & Poland, 1988) found similar results with a sample of 340 high school students: 40% of the students surveyed reported they had thought of suicide, while 11% reported a previous attempt. In addition, 51% reported that they knew someone who had attempted suicide, and 29% knew someone who had completed suicide. Friend (1988) reporting on the results of a survey of 11,419 8th- and 10th graders from 217 schools in 20 states found that 34% of them had seriously thought of suicide and 14% had tried it.

Davis (1985) has emphasized the unanimous agreement by researchers that the teenage suicide problem is underreported. Unreported attempts may outnumber reported ones by as much as 4:1. Davis commented after surveying available research,

> [I]n spite of a generally low rate of completions, given a high school population of 2000 children, it is predicated [that] a school psychologist could expect suicidal ideation in perhaps as high as 25 to 30% of the student body, suicide attempts by as many 50 students each year, and about one successfully completed suicide every 4 years. (1985, p. 314)

I first read this prediction several years ago and have found it to be an accurate prediction, if not an underestimate. *USA Today* (April 21, 1987) reported a survey of 500 teenagers indicating that 73% of the respondents had thought about suicide themselves and 70% knew someone who had attempted suicide. Leder (1987) has cited suicide as the second leading killer of teens, as noted in Chapter 1, and has also estimated that one in five teenagers are depressed. Ross (1985a) has estimated that at least 500,000 teenagers attempt suicide each year.

Berman (1985), in discussing the incidence of teen suicide, sounds a note of caution: He warns that in the rush to devote resources to the problem, we may be drawing conclusions about the rate of the increases too quickly. Berman comments,

> We have a significant public health problem with which to contend and develop appropriate and effective preventative strategies. The success of our efforts depends on a reasoned and scientific approach. Hyperbole and mis-education need not belong in that effort. (1985, p. 3)

At the National Conference on Youth Suicide, held in 1985, Livingston reported that suicide incidence per 100,000 in the 15–24 age range has increased from 4.1 in 1950 to 12.5 in 1980. This represents a 300% increase. School personnel need to be familiar with the concept of reporting suicides per 100,000 in the population. It is also important to recognize that school personnel might view a rate of 12.5 per 100,000 as unlikely to affect them: However, if a school district has 8,000 students in that age range, then 1 death a year could be predicted. The National Conference on Youth Suicide also stressed that at least 2 million high school students attempt suicide each year.

The conference further noted that suicidal-equivalent behaviors, such as substance usage, reckless behavior with cars and firearms, and eating disorders, were responsible for an additional 42,000 deaths in 1982 for the 15–24 age group. The conclusion was reached that 75% of the deaths nationally in this age group were related to self-destructive life styles. These figures have tremendous implications for what we attempt to teach students in the curriculum.

Government figures place the incidence of teen suicide at 5,000 deaths per year (Center for Disease Control, 1986). In 1987 a newscast reported figures in the 7,000–10,000 range for teenage suicides annually.

Boyd and Mościcki (1986) point out that the suicide rate in the United States has remained relatively stable, with the rate for youths increasing and the rate for adults declining. They also stress the dramatic increase in suicide death by firearms since 1970. Gun sales in this country have increased dramatically since the 1960s; in 1986, there were 75 guns for every 100 Americans. There is a high correlation between the availability of guns and the increase of youth suicide. Boyd and Mościcki stress the necessity to limit gun availability to reduce youth suicide.

Smith (1985) has addressed the question of the relationship between income level and suicide incidence, and notes that suicide incidence goes up with increased affluence.

Eyeman (1987) reports that the rate of suicide for the 5–14 age group increased from 0.1 per 100,000 in 1954 to 0.7 per 100,000 in 1984. The National Center for Health Statistics reported 137 suicides in the 10–14 age range for 1980. Eyeman reports that 40% of the adolescents who committed suicide had a history of suicide in the family, and 70% had alcohol in their blood. Eyeman stresses that the suicide rate for white males is the highest, with recent increases in the rate for black males and females; he also notes that females increasingly are using guns as a means of suicide.

Pfeffer (1986) has reported incidence figures of 28,542 suicides in the United States in 1982, with 200 in the 5–14 age group and 5,025 in the 15–24 age group. Pfeffer believes that the lower incidence in this 5–14 age group is related to stronger identification with the family, less abstract thinking resulting in less depression, and fewer feelings of loneliness.

Suicide is overall the seventh leading cause of death in the U.S. (McGinnis, 1987). McGinnis (1987) has stressed that suicide is moving up the public health priority list and that it must be approached as a public health issue. He comments that "overall improvements in the health of Americans tend to mask disturbing trends in the toll of death from suicide" (p. 18). Most threats to our health have declined with the exceptions of drug and alcohol abuse, homicide, and suicide. McGinnis has stressed that the government statistics showing 287,322 suicides in the United States from 1970 to 1980 (i.e., one suicide every 20 minutes) are staggering; nevertheless, they are an underestimate because medical examiners sometimes erroneously rule a suicide as a homicide or accident because of a variety of reasons. McGinnis cites a survey of medical examiners that estimated the number of reported suicides to be less than half the actual number.

The leading cause of death for teenagers is accidents, many of which involve automobiles and firearms. Obvious factors contributing to such accidents include substance usage and suicidal-equivalent behavior involving impaired judgment and recklessness. There are many single-car fatal automobile accidents in this country each year. Car accidents account for 37% of all deaths in the 15–24 age category, and it has been speculated that 25% of these deaths were intentional (Leder, 1987). I agree with the comments given above that the figures on youth suicide are staggering but undoubtedly a significant underestimate. The CDC's

(1986) report on youth suicide emphasizes that there is neither a common definition of suicide nor a set classification system, and some coroners do not classify a death as a suicide without a suicide note.

There appears to be growing agreement about the need for more suicide intervention in this country, but there is no national association to work on this problem as there are for other leading causes of death, such as heart and lung disease. These statistics lead me to believe that most of our population will somehow come into contact with a suicidal individual, and it is essential that we include education on this topic as part of school programs. A recent *USA Today* article (August 21, 1987) cited CDC estimates that suicides took 1.2 million years of potential life from their victims, based on a life expectancy of 65 years. Firearms accounted for 57% of the suicides reported, and white males lost the most years to suicide. Colt (1986) has pointed out that there are more suicides in the United States than murders.

It appears that it is nearly impossible to compile exact figures on the incidence of teenage suicide. It is also important to recognize that although much has been written about the incidence of teenage suicide, the actual incidence in our population increases with age, and those young people in the 20–24 age category are more at risk than those in the 15–19 age group. The latest government figures illustrating the rate of increase in the 5–14 category appear in Table 2.1; Table 2.2 displays the rise in incidence in the 15–24 category. The incidence of suicide among the young by race and sex is shown in Table 2.3.

School personnel need to know incidence figures that relate to the age group(s) they work with. As a general rule, suicide is rare under the age of 14. Government statistics show approximately 200 deaths a year in this age range. Common themes under the age of 14 are reckless behavior with

TABLE 2.1. Rise in Suicide Rate among Those Aged 5–14 in the United States, 1958 to 1982

Year	Rate per 100,000
1960	0.5
1970	0.5
1980	0.7
1982	0.9

Note. Adapted from *Suicide in the United States: 1958–1982* (p. 150) by the National Institute of Mental Health, 1985, Washington, DC: Government Printing Office.

TABLE 2.2. Rise in Suicides among Those Aged 15–24 in the United States, 1960 to 1980

Year	Number of deaths
1960	1,239
1970	3,128
1980	5,239

Note. Adapted from *Youth Suicide in the United States, 1970–1980* (p. 9) by the Centers for Disease Control, 1986, Atlanta: Author.

ropes or guns, climbing to high places, or running in front of cars. Texas had 10 suicides in 1980 by children under the age of 14; California led the nation with 15 (National Center for Health Statistics, 1980). We do need to take the suicidal statements of any student seriously, regardless of the student's age. The younger the child, probably the less clearly thought out is the plan and the less likely the child is to commit suicide, but we must take such children seriously. Table 2.1 shows that the incidence rate in the 10–14 age category has gone up significantly since 1970.

Tables 2.1 and 2.2 should be useful to school psychologists in dealing with administrators who are uncertain how much the incidence rate has increased. I have found it helpful to acknowledge that youth suicide was not a problem when most of our school administrators were in school, nor were administrators provided with coursework that emphasized this area; however, it is now essential that we recognize the problem, locate the most current incidence figures, and get to work on it. I also stress that the government figures simply cannot be ignored. These figures are not young people who *might* have committed suicide; these are the documented cases, and many others go unreported.

TABLE 2.3. Suicide Rates per 100,000 among the Young by Race and Sex, 1980

Race and sex	Ages 15–19	Ages 20–24
White males	15.0	27.8
White females	3.3	5.9
Black and other nonwhite males	7.5	20.9
Black and other nonwhite females	1.8	3.6

Note. Adapted from *Youth Suicide in the United States, 1970 to 1980* (p. 9) by the Centers for Disease Control, 1986, Atlanta: Author.

WHAT TYPE OF STUDENT COMMITS SUICIDE?

School personnel always ask many questions about the type of student who commits suicide. Does a certain race or sex have a higher incidence? White males definitely have the highest rate, as illustrated in Table 2.3. Suicide occurs across racial and ethnic boundaries, however; Smith (1985) and Eyeman (1987) have cited black males as the group whose suicide incidence has increased the most.

Schools also need to recognize the implications of the high incidence rate in the 20–24 age category. A suicide committed by a former student can still have a significant impact on the current student body. In one case I know of, a former student in this age range committed suicide; this had a great effect on his old high school, which his girlfriend and sister still attended.

Pfeffer (1986) has addressed the question of what the incidence will be in the year 2000. Her predictions for the various age groups show increases, possibly as high as 94% in the 15–19 category and 114% in the 20–24 category. It is difficult to make such predictions, but educators need to be aware that no dramatic decline in the incidence of youth suicide is expected. K. Smith (1988) states that the youth suicide rate peaked in 1985 and not 1977, as had earlier been reported.

Barrett (1985b) has addressed the question of why the suicide rates have not declined;

> I believe it is because efforts directed towards educating the public have been too limited in number and those intervention programs that have been implemented have often been too limited in scope. It is obvious that if the potentially suicidal youth [can] be identified and treatment can be given, the trend can be dramatically reversed. (p. 3)

School personnel also want to know where their particular state stands on the incidence of teenage suicide. Are there particular areas of the country where the incidence is higher? Table 2.4 addresses these questions. The CDC (1986) statistics show that the western United States had consistently higher suicide rates from 1970 to 1980 than the rest of the country. However, the difference in the rates by regions narrowed, and the rates for all regions increased over that period. Smith (1985) has cited increased mobility and weaker family roots in the western region as factors. It is also important to note the increased Indian population in western states, as there is documentation of increased suicide incidence among Native Americans (Eyeman, 1987; Smith, 1985). I think that looking at this data by state or geographical region is informative, but the important conclusion to be drawn is that suicide does occur in every state.

TABLE 2.4. Suicide Rates per 100,000 for All Persons 15–24 Years of Age by State of Residence, United States, 1980

8.6–12.1	12.2–15.7	15.8–19.3	19.4–22.9	23.0–26.5
Hawaii	Delaware	Florida	North Dakota	New Mexico
Nebraska	Texas	Colorado	Wyoming	Alaska
Maryland	Louisiana	Arizona		Nevada
Iowa	Washington	Montana		
New Jersey	California	Oregon		
Arkansas	Idaho	Vermont		
Illinois	Utah			
Indiana	South Dakota			
Kentucky	Minnesota			
Tennessee	Kansas			
North Carolina	Missouri			
Michigan	Oklahoma			
South Carolina	Ohio			
Georgia	Pennsylvania			
Alabama	West Virginia			
Mississippi	Virginia			
New York	Maine			
District of Columbia	Wisconsin			
Massachusetts				
Rhode Island				
Connecticut				
New Hampshire				

Note. Adapted from *Youth Suicide in the United States, 1970 to 1980* (p. 22) by the Centers for Disease Control, 1986, Atlanta: Author.

A review of the figures from the CDC (1986) shows an increase from 1970 to 1980 from 8.8 to 12.3 per 100,000 in the 15–24 category. There were 49,496 youth suicides during this period. The rate for persons aged 20–24 years of age was nearly twice the rate for persons aged 15–19. The increase was primarily due to the rising rate of suicide for males. Male suicides increased by 50% during this period, whereas female suicides increased by only 2%. The majority of male suicide victims were white (89.5%). The methods of suicide changed dramatically over this period, with suicide by firearms increasing and suicide by poisoning declining.

Two government agencies are working on the problem of youth suicide. The CDC and the National Institute of Mental Health have set the following goals: to document important trends and characteristics of youth suicide, and to implement strategies to decrease the suicide rate in the 15–24 age group to 11.0 by 1990. Among the primary strategies recommended are establishing comprehensive suicide intervention programs in the schools, and making young people more aware of where and how to get help through community agencies such as crisis centers.

SUMMARY

This chapter has discussed the incidence of teenage suicide. It is simply not possible to compile totally accurate figures of the incidence. All evidence indicates that government figures underestimate the problem. The incidence has increased dramatically in the last 20 years, and schools cannot simply stand by and wait for a suicide to occur. It is important for the schools to obtain the most recent information about trends and incidence. I have found it very helpful to assemble reports, data, and newspapers clippings to document this problem not only in my area but nationally. The CDC's 1986 report, which contains 71 pages of statistics, is also helpful.

Most school-based suicide intervention programs are developed in the aftermath of tragedy; this does not have to be the case. School personnel need to know that according to a conservative estimate, approximately 20 young people commit suicide each day in this country, and there are approximately 50–120 attempts for each completion (Smith & Crawford, 1986). This means that all who work in the schools will encounter this problem in some form or another. The implementation of an intervention program will only take place after we recognize that this problem can affect our schools and that we can take definite action to reduce the problem.

3

A Case Study

As I looked over my notes in preparation for writing this book, I realized how much of an impact this particular case had had on me and my efforts to work on suicide intervention in the schools. I have reported this case as realistically as I think is appropriate. It raises many of the questions that this book addresses. To be honest, I wish that I had known then what I now know about suicide intervention in the schools, although I believe that on the whole the case was handled appropriately.

SCHOOL DAY 1

My first notification of the suicide attempt of a high school boy was on a Friday morning. The principal called and informed me that the boy had shot himself after school on Thursday; he was in a coma, and the prognosis was not good. He had viewed a film on suicide in his sixth-period sociology class on Thursday. The teacher of that class was very upset, and the principal asked me to come and talk to her. My immediate reaction was one of panic and despair. I questioned whether I could help. I did not tell the principal this; instead, I said that I would be right there, although I wanted to go anywhere else that morning but to that school. It took me several interviews to get an accurate picture of what had happened.

A senior, B, had been depressed for some time and had talked with several friends about attempting suicide. His parents were divorced, and there were communication problems at home. The boy had no contact with his natural father, which resulted in feelings of loss and rejection. B had engaged in reckless behavior and, according to friends, had attempted suicide previously. His grades were relatively good, and he had many friends. He and his girlfriend were having difficulty and had recently broken up; the precipitating event may have been the perceived loss of the relationship with his girlfriend.

On the Thursday in question, B left school after viewing the first half of a made-for-television movie entitled *Silence of the Heart.* He located his girlfriend, who was in after-school detention. He got her attention by standing in the doorway of the classroom; he made eye contact with her, put a finger to his head, and walked away. He also put a note on her car that said, "Goodbye, you can't stop me this time!" B then went home and made one call to a female friend. Her father answered the phone and told her that B wanted to talk with her; she told her father to tell him that she would call him later. A few minutes later was too late. B shot himself in the head and was found by his younger brother when he came home from school.

My initial stop on Friday was at the principal's office. I made several specific suggestions to the principal, both orally and in written form. I still have those written suggestions, and the main points were as follows: (1) The school administrator should acknowledge what has happened, in order to dispel rumors; (2) both students and faculty should be allowed the opportunity to talk and should be given permission for a range of emotions; (3) networking was essential; and (4) the curriculum unit itself might be criticized by B's family, other parents, or the media.

I met with the teacher of the class and was very impressed with her. The teacher had very natural feelings of shock and disbelief. We talked about those feelings, and I found it helpful to share how I personally had been affected by suicide. The teacher had not been worried about B and had not detected any warning signs. We discussed the unit on suicide that she had put together, and I was impressed by it. A question that we had to address immediately was what to do with the sixth-period class that afternoon. I knew that she had to meet that class. We discussed the importance of acknowledging what had happened and giving the students permission for a range of emotions; we also agreed that it would be important for the teacher to model expression of emotions. In addition, we discussed the need to stress that B's problems were unique to him and that a suicide attempt was the result of long-standing, serious problems. We wanted to stress tactfully that we cared about him but that he must have had some very serious problems.

I was present when the students quietly filed into class that afternoon. The teacher did a good job of modeling expression of feelings and giving permission for discussion. I remember her saying that we just did not know what caused B to shoot himself, and she stressed that no problem could be that bad. She also emphasized the positive aspects of life and said that most bad things do work themselves out. The students asked a few questions, but they were mostly in a state of shock and denial. Everyone was very aware of the two empty chairs in the middle of the classroom; one belonged to B and the other to his girlfriend, who was at the hospital.

I found it helpful in establishing rapport to let the students know that I was a survivor of a suicide. I also said that I was the only person there who did not know B and that I was sorry I hadn't met him. I tried to prepare them for either his death or the possibility of lasting injury. I also mentioned that I knew that in a time of need, family members liked to receive cards and contacts from the close friends of their children. I discussed prayer as one additional concrete thing that the students could do.

One student asked whether they could see the rest of the made-for-television movie. The teacher and I agreed to show it. I did offer to talk individually with anyone who did not want to see the movie, and I also offered passes to the counselors' office. Everyone stayed to watch the conclusion of the movie. The second half of the movie showed a teenage boy wrestling with the guilt he felt at not recognizing the warning signs that his friend had given him. The boy decided to attempt suicide himself, but was stopped by his friends' parents. The ending of the movie was a very emotional one, but did leave a feeling of hope and showed the importance of intervention. The students seemed to get some sense of closure from watching the movie.

Several students were crying when school ended for the day. The general tone of their comments were that they could not believe what had happened, nor did they believe that seeing the movie was the cause of B's suicide attempt. They were very upset and puzzled by the attempt. After the departure of the students, I complimented the teacher on how she had handled the situation. She indicated that she wanted to call B's mother and stepfather or go to their house, and asked what I thought of that idea. I said that this would be difficult but was definitely a very appropriate thing to do. I also mentioned that I knew that one of the school counselors had been to the hospital to see the parents, and that reaching out to parents at a time of need was very commendable and appropriate for school personnel to do. I told the teacher that I would see her Monday, and went to see the principal to give him feedback on how the sixth-period class had gone.

The principal was relieved that the class had gone as well as could be expected. I told him that I was very impressed with the teacher and the way in which she had handled the situation. We agreed that I would return on Monday morning, and he thanked me profusely for my assistance. I thanked him in turn for his willingness to deal directly with the situation. I felt very drained and saddened by the almost certain death of the young man, but I also felt positive about my response; I had not panicked or become so grief-stricken as to be ineffective.

On Sunday, I was notified of another suicide attempt. A female student in the same grade as B had attempted carbon monoxide poisoning. The girl had started the engine of her car in the garage with the door shut. She passed out and fell against the horn; a neighbor heard the horn and rescued her. She was hospitalized, but was in stable condition, and a complete recovery was expected. I immediately called the principal and told him what had happened. We agreed to meet at school the next morning with his administrative and counseling team. He indicated that he would use his "calling tree" to inform his administrative and counseling team. This prior knowledge allowed us all to give thought to how we could proceed.

SCHOOL DAY 2

A counselor at the meeting on Monday morning immediately announced that there had been one more attempt on Sunday. A freshman boy had ingested pills and had been rushed to the hospital, where his stomach was pumped; he was now okay. He did not know B or the girl who had attempted suicide, but had heard of their attempts. B was still in a coma. It was obvious that all concerned were looking to me to provide leadership.

My recommendations were similar to those I had given on Friday. I felt that we needed to control rumors, allow opportunities for students to talk about their feelings, and continue our networking efforts. I also stated that we might also receive attention from the news media. I advised against any kind of large-scale assembly. We all recognized the contagion effect. We decided to reach all students by means of classroom presentations and elected to use English classes, as every student in the school had to take English. The principal sent for all English team leaders.

I provided the team leaders with a brief overview of crisis theory and the stages of the grief process. I also outlined seven major points, which were included in the presentation to all English classes:

1. Students were given the facts, and rumors were dispelled.
2. The teachers modeled expression of feelings and gave the students permission to talk about their feelings. (Many of the English teachers also gave students the opportunities to express their feelings through their writing.)
3. The positive aspects of life were emphasized. It was emphasized that the faculty cared about the students.
4. The teachers avoided romanticizing or glorifying suicide.

5. It was emphasized that these young people who had attempted suicide had unique, long-standing problems.

6. Teachers emphasized the warning signs of suicide and noted that the intervention of a friend could mean the difference between life and death. Confidentiality was addressed, and examples were given to illustrate that students should not keep secrets about suicidal behavior. The local crisis hotline number was provided.

7. Teachers informed students that counselors and psychologists were available each period and after school.

This format effectively reached all 2,700 students in the high school. It did result in large numbers of students requesting counseling, and it also resulted in many papers depicting sadness and focusing on suicide, which were brought to my attention.

Several other strategies were outlined in our administrative meeting. A psychologist was designated to follow B's class schedule to help his teachers answer questions and discuss the events of the past few days. In addition, counselors and psychologists concentrated on networking activities. All students known to be suicidal were counseled, and teachers were instructed that if they knew of anyone who had previously attempted suicide, they should contact a counselor. All who counseled with students kept notes, and a list was compiled of who was seen and by whom. Parents were notified if we were concerned about their son or daughter. "No-suicide" contracts were signed by a number of students. Group sessions were held during each period of the school day to accommodate the large number of grieving students; these sessions were in addition to individual counseling. Finally, a follow-up meeting for the administrative and counseling team was held, and a faculty meeting was scheduled for the next day. These strategies set the course of action not only for the next few hours, but for the next several days. Everyone had a role to play, and lines of communication were clarified.

One of the immediate concerns of mine was what to do with the many papers discussing suicide. I had not anticipated that so many students would want to express themselves in writing. I devised a scale to rate the suicidal risk of the students based on their papers, in order to determine which students needed attention first. Each paper was read by two raters. Something that surprised me was that several English teachers felt that they were violating the confidentiality of the students by letting someone else read their papers. I emphasized that it was absolutely essential that we not keep secrets about suicidal behavior.

A handout on adolescent suicide prevention was distributed to all faculty members. The handout emphasized what teachers should look for to detect suicidal behavior and how to respond to suicidal students. The handout, entitled "Teenage Suicide Prevention Tips" (Schindler & Poland, 1985), appears as Appendix A of this book. Several teachers commented that they were grateful to have it.

Counselors and psychologists spent Monday talking with students individually or in groups. Networking efforts resulted in a group of seniors starting a telephone network to assist those students who were the closest to B. Several of the friends who were the closest to B were not in school; they were at the hospital. School counselors kept in touch with them by telephone. Some students were at school, but wanted to leave and go to the hospital. We encouraged them to stay at school; however, if their parents gave them permission to leave school, then we allowed them to do so. We called their parents with the students present for clarification. This also gave us an opportunity to discuss with parents how they could help their son or daughter. A common parental concern was that their children were not confiding enough in them. Many parents were scared and uncertain how to approach their children. One mother commented, "B was my son's close friend, and this is the worst thing that has ever happened to my son." I recommended that parents take a direct approach and bring up the events of the past few days. I also recommended that parents be honest about their own feelings and fears. It was also important for parents to increase their availability to their children; in some cases, I recommended increased supervision.

Many students sought help for their friends who were suicidal. Some of the barriers to telling adults were down, and students were willing to speak up and get help for their friend. As a result, one more suicide attempt came to our attention: Another girl had taken pills in an attempt to end her life. She, like the boy who had taken pills on Sunday, was now okay. A counselor and I met with the ninth-grade girl. She said that she did not know B, but had heard of his attempt and decided to follow through on her earlier plans to kill herself. She appeared very lonely and was very distressed about her natural father, who had totally rejected her. She was also very upset about her appearance, as she needed extensive dental work. She signed a no-suicide contract and responded well to the news that her mother would be called and asked to come to the school to talk with us. Her mother was very cooperative and agreed to follow through on our referral to a private psychologist. A phone call 2 days later was necessary to encourage the mother to actually make an appointment. She commented that she thought that her daughter seemed better and that help was no longer needed. I told her that I thought otherwise.

School was out on Monday much too quickly, and we had not done all that we wanted to. A meeting was held after school. The English team leaders reported on how things had gone in all the English classes. It was felt that students had needed an opportunity to talk it out and had appreciated getting the facts. Rumors of suicide pacts had been widespread, especially a rumor that B and his girlfriend had both attempted suicide. I suggested that a follow-up discussion be conducted the next few days and that a resumption of regular academic activities be gradual. An update on B's medical condition was not encouraging. A few students had been in to see him and were very distressed at all the bandages and the swelling. He was still in a coma, although his girlfriend claimed that he had squeezed her hand.

The counseling staff gave an update on the three additional suicide attempts. Plans were made to continue the group sessions, which, as mentioned above, were open to everyone each period of the school day. There was much discussion of individual students about whom staff members were concerned. I had again visited with the teacher of B's sixth-period class after school, and reported that she was "hanging in there." She had visited with B's parents, and they had told her that they did not think that a movie caused him to shoot himself.

SCHOOL DAY 3

Tuesday brought more of the same, with much discussion of suicide throughout the school. A fourth student had attempted suicide by turning on the gas at home, but changed her mind and turned off the gas. She did not know any of the other students personally, but had heard of their attempts. Her mother was cooperative; however, she had no insurance to cover counseling and stated that she couldn't afford to pay for it. I made an appointment for her with a private practitioner and arranged for the district to pay for a consultation.

A counselor brought me the news that a former student had been killed in a car accident the night before and that his girlfriend was a current student. Assistance and support were provided to her.

One counselor also consulted with me about a student who was reported to be suicidal and could not be located. The school was searched, and he was not found. His parents were notified; they found him in the neighborhood and brought him back to school. He was depressed, but had no plan to commit suicide.

The local news media began to call on this day. The principal and I worked closely with the public information director. It was decided that I would do the interviews. I had done interviews a few times before about teenage suicide; however, this time was different because the problem was a specific outbreak of suicide attempts with which I was working, not a general issue. I agreed to a television interview, but I did ask a few questions about what approach the reporter was going to take. The reporter emphasized that he would be asking about what the school was doing and how students and faculty were coping with this outbreak of teen suicide. I closeted myself in an office, rehearsed answers to each of those questions (and others that I anticipated) aloud, and prayed that I wouldn't be too nervous as I awaited the mobile camera. I knew that what would appear on the air would be brief and that I needed to be concise and to the point in my comments.

The television reporter arrived and was friendly. I asked how his station had heard of the story, and he indicated that a parent had called the news desk to report several suicide attempts among students from the high school. I knew that I could not release any private information about any of these students or their families. My strategy was to talk in general about the problem and to stress that our district was prepared to deal with it. The reporter's first question was "How do you feel about this young boy who is in a coma and not expected to live?" That one caught me off guard, but I recovered quickly to say that I was very saddened. He then gave me several opportunities to stress all that we had done in the past several days. I also was able to mention that the district had a suicide prevention program, which had been in operation for 4 years. The reporter went on to discuss the several attempts following the attempt by B. Several of his details were inaccurate, and he referred to an attempt a month previously that I knew nothing about, but I did not correct him. The reporter took lots of pictures of the school and approached several teachers for comments. The teachers referred him to the principal, and I don't believe that he was allowed to talk to any students.

There were two more interview requests. I was live on the air for several minutes on local news radio, and I did an interview for the Associated Press. The radio interview went reasonably well, and I was able to discuss teenage suicide in general and what could be done about it. The reporter for the Associated Press was very interested in the story because he thought it was a suicide pact. He noticeably lost interest when I clarified that this was not the case. I asked where this story might be printed, and the reporter indicated that it could be in every newspaper or none.

A faculty meeting was held after school. I will never forget standing up in front of the entire faculty of 150. I had watched them enter the auditorium, and it seemed as if the entire weight of teenage suicide was on their shoulders. The principal gave them an update. B's condition was essentially the same: He was in a coma and was not expected to live. There had now been four other suicide attempts by students, but all were okay. A former student had been killed in a car accident. Three interviews had been granted to the media. The principal then asked me to share with the faculty what we had been doing, and I shared with them the strategy that we were following. I emphasized strongly that teenage suicide was a societal problem and that these students had long-standing personal problems. Teenage suicide was not just our high school's problems. I discussed all of the prevention efforts that we had made, and specifically emphasized the teachers' role and how that had helped and could continue to help. In addition, I mentioned and debunked the most important myths on the subject—the myths that "talking about it makes it worse" and that a suicidal person truly wants to die and cannot be stopped. I also addressed the question of how much effect watching the movie on teen suicide had had on B. I said that in my opinion, it had played a very small role. I tried to be as positive as possible, citing our preparation, our resources, and our plan of action. I closed with a statement of hope that things would improve.

SCHOOL DAY 4

The first news that I heard when I arrived at school on Wednesday was that B had died the previous evening. I received this news with sadness, although I had been expecting it. I would never meet this boy about whom I now knew so much after talking to so many of his friends and teachers. I wondered whether I would ever meet his parents.

The school openly and honestly acknowledged B's death through small-group announcements and discussion. His close friends returned to school. It was announced that B's funeral would be the following day; the principal designated several staff members to represent the school. Many students discussed with us whether or not they should attend the funeral. Our position was that this decision was for them and their parents to make. There would be no penalty for missing school to attend the funeral. I encouraged those who were really close to him to go and those who were not close friends to stay in school.

Most students were coping well and were prepared for B's death. There seemed to be a sense of closure to a very difficult and emotional chapter as the entire school dealt with the reality of teen suicide. Individuals' personal life history, their closeness to B, and their knowledge of B's intentions affected their ability to cope. The students we were the most concerned about were his girlfriend and the girl he had tried to call shortly before he shot himself. Neither had attended school since the incident; however, a school counselor had talked with each of them and their families daily. Both girls began private counseling at our recommendation. There were no new reports of suicide attempts.

Most of the faculty members at the school had watched the previous evening's local newscast, which showed the interview with me. Many people complimented me on it, and I was told that a tape was in the principal's office if I wished to view it. The general theme of the feature was how a local community was dealing with teen suicide. The district was portrayed as concerned and prepared and as having approached the problem directly and openly. The warning signs and sources of help were included in the broadcast. I will never forget the closing statement that the reporter made. He said that our school district believed that more dialogue on teen suicide was needed, but that not everyone agreed with this approach. I felt encouraged that the interview had gone as well as it had. The principal, the public information director, and the superintendent were very complimentary.

I received a phone call from a parent that brought me back down to earth. Her opening statement was this: "How dare you use my daughter's name on television as someone who had attempted suicide!" I was really taken aback, as I did not know her or her daughter and certainly did not use anyone's name. I assured her that I had not mentioned names on the broadcast, and was able to figure out that her daughter must have been the student the reporter had mentioned as having attempted suicide a month earlier. This entire incident was news to me, and I said so. I offered to assist her daughter in any way that I could. She declined my offer and hung up without even so much as an apology. I have given this phone call a lot of thought. I think that this mother's reaction illustrates the fear, uncertainty, and shame that many parents feel when their children attempt suicide. This mother was more interested in covering up the incident than in getting help for her child. I wish that we could change these attitudes, and, yes, I do believe that more dialogue on the topic does help.

The media account of this contagion situation was manageable. Had there been a second death, things would have undoubtedly been different. There was no more news coverage other than B's obituary, which appeared in the paper with no mention of the cause of death.

SCHOOL DAY 5

Students and faculty returned from the funeral on Thursday and commented on how nice it had been. Networking efforts continued as counselors and psychologists worked with students. There was much less talk about teen suicide, and teachers reported that classes were returning to normal. I visited again with the teacher of B's sixth-period class. She was very aware that it was a week ago since the incident had taken place.

There were no more suicide attempts. That afternoon a beautiful fruit basket arrived at the psychological services department from the staff at the high school, thanking us for all our assistance. It was appreciated.

SCHOOL DAY 6

Counselors continued to work with students on Friday. The additional psychologists who had been pulled in to help at the high school were released to work elsewhere. One thing that we were thankful for was that the problem had not spread to any of our other high schools. A follow-up strategy was outlined that involved psychologists' calling back to check on students that were at risk. The intent was to return all counseling and monitoring to the staff members regularly assigned to the school. I planned to continue to check on the sixth-period teacher to see how she was doing. I remained on the campus until school was out. Everyone seemed positive, and the school climate appeared normal. It had been a long week.

POSTSCRIPT

I received a call from the superintendent 2 weeks later, indicating that B's parents had asked to view the movie he had seen. The superintendent said that he felt I should be the one to show it to them. I agreed to do so, but with much trepidation. I wondered what their motives were. Were they thinking of suing us? I also knew that I wanted to involve a curriculum director in this process.

I had had nothing to do with the selection of that movie, nor was I that knowledgeable about the curriculum and suicide prevention. Our efforts up to that point had concentrated on intervention—detecting suicidal behavior, assessing its severity level, and notifying parents. The superintendent agreed that it was a good idea to involve the curriculum director. The director agreed to view the film, and we made an appointment to prepare for our conference with B's parents. I was very impressed with the curriculum director. One of the first things that I shared with him was my personal experience with suicide. He then shared with me that there had also been a suicide in his family. In addition, we discussed whether or not to include the teacher. The curriculum director had met with the teacher and had received a detailed overview of the unit. We agreed not to include the teacher, primarily because we did not want the group to be large.

B's mother, stepfather, younger brother, and grandfather attended the conference. We opened the conference by offering our condolences to the family. I remember saying that I knew this would be difficult for all of us, and the director and I both shared our personal experiences with suicide. Rapport was thus established, as all present had a common bond.

We watched the movie in its entirety. There were many tears for each of us. Tears seemed to run continually down the cheeks of B's grandfather. It took several minutes after the movie ended for each person to gain his or her composure. The parents made several comments. The mother commented that she remembered when this movie was on television; she had thought about watching it but hadn't. She also stated that she knew that the school district had provided evening sessions to inform parents about clues to teen suicide. She had not attended any of these sessions, nor had she read the article in her *Reader's Digest* on the subject. She had meant to learn more about this subject, but she just didn't think that she needed to. She and her husband had not known that B had attempted suicide previously. They also had not thought he knew where they kept a pistol for protection. The parents' comments could be summarized by the statement that they didn't think that suicide could ever happen to them. They learned about suicide too late. They told us that if we could help anyone learn anything from their son's death through sharing information about what happened, we should feel free to do so. They hoped other parents would not have to go through what they had.

The grandfather asked several questions. He wanted to know about the discussion that was held with students before the movie was shown, he also asked at what point the movie was stopped after the first day, and how much discussion time there was the first day. He seemed satisfied with our answers. There was no criticism of the unit on suicide prevention and no criticism of the movie. Again, the general tone of the discussion was that perhaps if the parents had known more about suicide prevention, this tragedy could have been prevented. The younger brother was very quiet throughout and was continually comforted by his parents and grandfather. The family members thanked us for our time and our efforts to prevent teen suicide, and especially for our efforts to help B's friends. The director and I discussed the conference and felt that it had gone well. It was a tragedy, but we all had to go on and try to learn from it. We both liked the family members and empathized with them.

The counseling team leader at B's high school put together an overview of the events for the superintendent and principal. The overview was very complimentary toward the psychological services department and stressed that the entire staff of the high school had responded in a caring and cooperative manner. Parents were very appreciative of the school's efforts, and the members of the senior class pulled together to try to help one another. Students also received guidance to memorialize B in an appropriate manner through a scholarship fund, and not through any dedication of an event or publication or through a lasting memorial at the school.

Assistant principals at the high school approached me the next fall concerning a seminar for student leaders. The school had many clubs and organizations, and their respective officers were invited to participate in a leadership seminar. They outlined goals for the year, one of which was to prevent teenage suicide by establishing their own crisis hotline. The students wanted me to help with this project. I agreed to help, but had reservations about the project. I spoke with a former crisis hotline staff member with whom I now worked, and we agreed to meet with the students. The seminar involved approximately 60 students. We provided them with lots of information about teen suicide and practical examples of what they could do, but we also tried to talk them out of creating their own hotline. We attempted to channel their efforts toward supporting the existing local hotline; those students over 18 years of age could be trained as volunteers, and those under 18 could disseminate information about the hotline or raise funds to help support it. The students were adamant that they wanted to try an after-school hotline. We agreed to organize one and to train the students who would answer the phones.

The principal expressed some reservations, but was reassured by knowing that counselors and psychologists would be present to assist with the calls. Fifteen students went through the 6-hour training session. One afternoon from 3 P.M. until 9 P.M. was designated as the school "Crisis Helpline." There were not very many calls, and none were of serious nature. I believe that the existence of the activity was underpublicized. I do view the activity as very positive, because those students who received the training learned a great deal, and I feel that they are well prepared to assist a suicidal person in the future.

I tried to keep in touch with B's friends the next year, though this was difficult because they had all graduated. I was saddened to hear that his girlfriend attempted suicide on his birthday. She survived, and the family took her back to counseling. I was also approached by the mother of another girl to whom B had been close, who asked my advice on how to help her daughter. She stated that B's death was still very difficult for her daughter. Her daughter often looked at a picture B had given her shortly before his suicide. The picture showed him with his eyes closed, and the girl wondered whether that was a clue to his plans. I gave the mother a few suggestions and referral sources, one of which was the local survivors' group. Assistance follow-up was provided to B's brother and several younger neighbors.

The counseling and administration team made an interesting statement when another boy shot himself a year later: "We know what to do this time, and we have confidence that we can proceed and help our students and faculty deal with this." They had learned much from B's suicide and the events that surrounded it. B's case was very complex, involving curriculum issues and a contagion situation. The news media were also involved, and the school and the community were affected. This case example raises many questions about teen suicide. The remainder of this book attempts to provide practical guidelines for suicide intervention in the schools.

4

Forces and Factors in Teen Suicide

School personnel want to know why the incidence of teenage suicide has increased. What causes a teenager to commit suicide? Are young people of a certain age group, personality type, or family background more likely than others to attempt suicide? Are handicapped students more at risk than students who are not handicapped? What effect does the music that teenagers listen to have on suicide rates? What about the media attention to teen suicide through national news coverage? Do made-for-television movies help promote public awareness that results in a reduction of suicide rates, or do these movies cause more suicides? Are there certain times of the year that teenagers are more likely to turn to suicide? What part do academic and competitive pressures in our society play? What part does the breakdown of the family unit, which has resulted in many one-parent families and frequent movement, play in teen suicide? Is there a mystic or romantic aspect to teenage suicide? What effect do motion pictures like *The Deer Hunter*, which graphically depict suicide, have on teenagers? How do teenagers respond when someone in their family models suicide as a way of coping with problems? Are teenagers likely to try suicide in the wake of a suicide by another teen through a "contagion effect"? Do teenagers actually express their suicidal thoughts through tragic essays? How much influence do drugs and alcohol have on the suicide of young people? Do teenagers actually imagine the impact of their own death on their loved ones and friends? What precipitating events trigger a suicide attempt? Are runaway adolescents at greater risk of attempting suicide? Can teenage suicide be explained by looking only at depression? How do suicidal adolescents differ from suicidal adults? Do teenagers understand the finality of death? Do they sometimes get so heavily involved in fantasy games such as "Dungeons and Dragons" that they cannot separate themselves from the games? Are more teenagers using firearms in an attempt to take their lives?

These questions illustrate many of the forces and factors that affect teenage suicide. The recognition of these factors will assist school personnel in their prevention efforts. I have been asked by school personnel on many occasions, "What causes teen suicide?" There is no absolute answer. Leder (1987) discusses as many as 15 causation factors. The various sections into which this chapter is divided illustrate the variety of possible forces and factors. There has been a national emphasis on identifying these forces and factors. The Office of the Inspector General (OIG), a division of the U.S. Department of Health and Human Services, conducted an inspection of youth suicide in the mid-1980s. The report of this inspection (OIG, 1986) found increases during this period in the following: (1) The number of very young attempters (aged 10 and under); (2) suicidal ideation among youths of all ages; (3) multiple forms of self-destructive behavior; and (4) a sense of futility among youths. Family problems were cited by more than half of the respondents as contributing to youth suicide. Family support was viewed as the key to treatment and a successful outcome. One-third of the suicidal youths interviewed were the victims of physical and/or sexual abuse.

FAMILY FACTORS

Many researchers have cited factors in youth suicide that relate to the breakdown of the family. The roots of the problem seem to be in the family. Youth suicide is the result both of long-standing problems and of a particular situation that an adolescent cannot face or cannot see a solution to. Explaining the increase in youth suicide is difficult. Heckler (1985) has emphasized such factors as stress, pressure, drug and alcohol use, divorce, and legal problems. Factors discussed by Davis (1985), include psychosis or personal disorganization, a wish for self-homicide, retaliation for abandonment, blackmail, manipulation, and a wish to rejoin a lost love object.

Looney, Oldham, Clamman, Crumley, and Walker (1985) found no clear-cut cause, but cited depression and other mental disorders in combination with family discord and personal and sociocultural factors. Peck et al. (1985) found that 90% of suicidal teens felt that their parents did not understand them. Communication problems have been cited by Johnson and Maile (1987) as primary causation factors. Coleman (1987a) has stated that the average parent spends only 7 minutes a week communicating with his or her teenager. Nelson, Farberow, and Litman (1987) describe the California Department of Mental Health study on causation factors. The study found that both intrapersonal and interpersonal problems contributed to youth suicide. Intrapersonal problems were in the areas of general stress, low self-esteem, family instability, communication problems with parents, and feelings of hopelessness and depression. Interpersonal factors were substance use, school problems, and peer problems. The question of school difficulty has also been addressed by Peck (1985), who found that 50% of youth suicide victims had a learning disability. Guetzloe (1988) cites a number of studies finding that disproportionate numbers of special education students have committed suicide.

Smith (1985) has emphasized the role of self-esteem and stress. Coleman (1987a) notes that losses can build up, resulting in a feeling of hopelessness. Other causes listed by Leder (1987) include blocked communication with parents, lack of bonding between parents and child, and role reversal (i.e., situations in which the child is forced to assume too much responsibility). Garfinkel (1986) stresses the contribution of family pathology. Withers and Kaplan (1987) emphasize family disruption, a history of madadaptive behavior, and the presence of depression. These authors found two-thirds of the suicidal youths they studied to be depressed.

By contrast, Garland (1987) emphasizes that we should not concentrate solely on depression as a causation factor, and stresses the role of antisocial behavior, substance use, and family history. Shaffer (1988) has summarized autopsy studies of youths who committed suicide; he notes that most of these suicides were impulsive acts, carried out when the youths were either enraged, intoxicated, or in a state of terror. Hendin (1987), in summarizing earlier research searching for causation factors, concludes that suicidal youngsters are often alienated from their parents early in their childhood and display attitudes of resistance and hostility in response to feeling rejected. Their feelings are likely to be expressed through reckless behavior and drug/alcohol usage. Hendin reports that some parents are not emotionally involved with their children; the message conveyed to these children is a feeling of not being wanted or needed in the family. Hendin has also examined the question of serotonin levels in young people who make violent suicide attempts, and has found that low serotonin levels are present in some cases.

Withers and Kaplan (1987) found in their study that the characteristics most often exhibited by adolescents in the year prior to their suicide attempts were alcohol use, drug usage, and rebellion toward authority. Only one-tenth of their sample came from harmonious families. They concluded that these teenagers were simply not receiving adequate family support.

Eyeman (1987) stresses that suicidal adolescents are not good at facing problems, nor are they adept at expressing their emotions. These adolescents may attempt suicide in order to avoid facing a frustrating situation.

Johnson and Maile (1987) list as causation factors competition, family disarray, increased divorce rates, both parents working, an inability to handle stress and anger, lack of adequate role models, and substance abuse. They review the work of Jacobs (1971), who has listed the following prerequisites for adolescent suicide. First, the problem is viewed as unsolvable and as one of a series of continuing problems. Second, suicide is viewed as the *only* answer, and this decision is made in isolation. Finally, the barrier of suicide as wrong is dealt with through viewing the problem as unsolvable and not of the adolescent's making.

Pfeffer (1986) has discussed the suicidal motives of children and the role that fantasy plays. Pfeffer emphasizes that suicidal fantasies provide the reasons for suicidal actions. The most common fantasy wishes are to die, to kill, to be rescued, or to escape from an intolerable situation. Other common fantasies are to be killed, to punish others, to achieve a peaceful state, or to rejoin a loved one. However, Pfeffer also stresses that suicidal fantasies alone do not lead to suicidal behavior. There must also be a breakdown in ego functioning in combination with stressors that result in painful helplessness feelings.

Toolan (1975) has classified youth suicide attempts into four categories: anger at another, attempt to manipulate, a signal of distress, and a reaction to personal disintegration.

The characteristics of families with suicidal potential have been addressed by Richman (1986). Richman lists seven major factors:

1. Necessary changes are not accepted.
2. Interpersonal failures result in role confusion and conflict.
3. Family structure is dysfunctional or disturbed.
4. Family relationships are confused, symbiotic, or double-binding.
5. The family has a pattern of emotional difficulty.
6. Communication problems exist.
7. Crises are not tolerated.

Richman pays special attention to the close association between separation and death. The suicidal person is often isolated within the family and discouraged from forming relationships outside of the family.

Family factors related to youth suicide cited by Eyeman (1987) include a history of affective disorder; previous suicide in the family; alcohol abuse in one or both parents; loss of a parent through death, separation, or divorce; physical or sexual abuse; family violence; an emphasis on high achievement; separation difficulty; and ineffective family patterns of managing stress. Similar factors are cited by Pfeffer (1986), who notes that suicidal children have a history of stress and loss in their families, coupled with a pattern of instability, drug/alcohol usage, and family violence. Suicidal children are also sometimes either consciously or unconsciously given the message that they are "expendable." Other disturbed family patterns include symbiotic relationships, inflexible family systems, severe marital conflicts, and parents who project their own unacceptable feelings onto the suicidal child.

Davis (1985) has discussed seven motives for suicide among adolescents. The most common is the "cry for help." The types are outlined below:

1. Psychosis or personality disorganization.
2. Self-homicide, which is characterized by intense rage at others that is directed at the self.
3. Retaliation for real or imagined abandonment.
4. Blackmail or manipulation in order to get treated better.
5. Rejoining a powerful lost love object.
6. Atonement for unpardonable sins.
7. A cry for help.

PRECIPITATING EVENTS

Family factors and the individual young person's history appear to set the stage for a suicide attempt. In addition, however, Brown (1987) notes that an event or loss can be the "straw that broke the camel's back" and can cause a young person to follow through on a suicide attempt. A report by the Indiana State Board of Health (1985) examined the precipitating events that led to suicide attempts in that state. The problem involved parents 52% of the time; 30% of the time it involved the opposite sex; 16% of the time it involved siblings; and 15% of the time it involved peers. Porter (1985) reported that 55% of suicide completers had recently experienced the death of a friend or relative. Shaffer (1988) emphasizes that suicidal teens are generally responding to an acute crisis, which most often involves discipline incidents, loss of face with peers, or arguments with parents. Eyeman (1987) has listed the most common stressors experienced by adolescents who attempt suicide as follows:

• Breakup with boyfriend or girlfriend
• Trouble with sibling
• Change in parents' finances
• Divorce
• Loss of a friend

- Trouble with a teacher
- Change of school
- Injury or illness
- Failing grades
- Increased arguments with friends

An example of a precipitating event was provided by a student who commented to me, "When I was expelled from school, I just couldn't take that. It was so bad, it just kept eating away at me, so I drove my car into a bridge." The most common precipitating event that I have seen has been the breakup of a relationship with a boyfriend or girlfriend. This leads to feelings of rejection, hopelessness, and the thought that "I can't go on without him [her]." Some irrational thoughts also surface along the lines of "I will never have another boyfriend [girlfriend]."

We must be careful not to minimize adolescents' intense emotions concerning attachments to boyfriends or girlfriends. It is also vitally important to pay attention to substance use and the availability of firearms. I have seen the following pattern numerous times: An adolescent with a personal and family history indicative of suicidal potential experiences a precipitating event; the young person then uses drugs or alcohol and suddenly takes out a firearm that is accessible. Tragedy is often the result. I think that the point made by Brown (1987) about not minimizing the impact that an event might have on an adolescent is a very important one. It is not the adult's perception of the event that is important; it is the adolescent's perception.

A survey of 500 teenagers in *USA Today* (April 21, 1987) found that the reason most often given for contemplating suicide was problems with parents. Other reasons were not being able to live up to others' expectations, loneliness, boyfriend/girlfriend problems, and concern about appearance.

Another source of stress for young people is frequent moves. It is not unusual for suicidal youths to have moved frequently. Barrett (1985b) has stressed that parents often underestimate the effects of moves on their children. The school can be very helpful in recognizing how hard a move is on an adolescent. Various activities should be planned for newcomers. One counselor tried the buddy system of matching a new student with a student of the same age, who was not new to the school. This match seemed to help only for a short time, however. The approach has now been changed to providing activities where all the new students meet one another.

DEPRESSION

Leder (1987) states that one-fifth of all teenagers are depressed. What part does depression play in the suicide attempt of a teenager? Does depression alone explain teenage suicide? Young people under the age of 18 comprise 20% of those hospitalized for depression (Porter, 1985). Pfeffer (1986) has stressed the significant association between affective disorders and suicidal behavior for both children and adults, and notes that depression is also a specific risk factor for suicide. Several researchers have emphasized that depression alone does not account for all suicidal behavior and that conduct-disordered adolescents may also be at risk of attempting suicide (Eyeman, 1987; Shaffer, 1988).

Davis (1985) discusses the Freudian view of suicide, which stresses depression as the cornerstone of suicidal behavior; he comments that "not all suicides can be understood from this perspective" (p. 317). There are indications that the majority of suicidal children are depressed, but not every depressed child is suicidal, nor is every suicidal child depressed.

Historically, there has been some disagreement about the existence of depression in children. Stark (1987) stresses that depression in a child under the age of 10 is very rare and is usually the result of extreme environmental problems and psychopathology in the family. By contrast, Barrett (1985b) feels that depression in children has been overlooked and that the notion that children do not get depressed is not true. Pfeffer (1986) has outlined three different viewpoints concerning depression and children: (1) Depressed children do not exist; (2) depressed children do exist, but symptoms mask their depression; and (3) depressed children exist, but with unique symptoms in addition to those exhibited by depressed adults. Pfeffer concludes that there is a consensus that depression in childhood exists as a psychiatric disorder.

The most recent criteria for diagnosing childhood depression are described in the revised third edition of the *Diagnostic and Statistical Manual of Mental Disorders* (DSM-III-R; American Psychiatric Association, 1987). Stark (1987) has estimated that between 4.5% and 14% of the children and adolescents who comprise the school population can be diagnosed as depressed according to the DSM-III-R criteria. The types of depression listed in the DSM-III-R include Major Depressive Disorder, Dysthymic Disorder, and Adjustment Disorder with Depressive Features.

An instrument recommended by both Pfeffer (1986) and Stark (1987) for assessing depression in childhood is the Schedule for Affective Disorder and Schizophrenia for School-Age Children—Present Episode (Kiddie-SADS-P). The instrument, which was developed by Chambers, Puig-Antich, and Tabrizi in 1978, is appropriate for children from 6 to 16 years of age and consists of a structured interview that thoroughly assesses the emotional state of the child. The interview takes approximately 2 hours with a depressed child.

Depression is a significant factor in teen suicide. Withers and Kaplan (1987) have stressed the need for school personnel to be sensitized to the symptoms of depression; they found two-thirds of the young people in their sample who had attempted suicide to be depressed. School personnel should be alert for physical and emotional signs of depression in children. The Indiana State Board of Health (1985) stated that 50% of depressed children admitted to having thoughts of hurting themselves, and stressed that depression must be distinguished from the normal mood swings of adolescence. The duration and intensity of the symptoms are the key to that distinction. The major symptoms of depression are as follows:

- Withdrawal from friends and activities
- Loss of joy in life and a bleak outlook for the future
- Changes in sleeping and eating habits
- Risk-taking or reckless behavior
- Preoccupation with death
- Increased somatic complaints
- Concentration problems with regard to school work
- Frequent mood changes
- Uncharacteristic emotional or rebellious outbursts
- Low self-esteem and lack of confidence in abilities and decision-making capabilities
- Significant weight loss or gain
- Decreased attention to physical appearance

SUBSTANCE ABUSE

At least 50% of the time, adolescents who attempt or complete suicide are under the influence of alcohol or drugs (Porter, 1985). Johnson and Maile (1987), reviewing the literature in this area, find unanimous agreement concerning the importance of this factor in teen suicide. And Davis, Sandoval, and Wilson (1988) suggest that major substance abuse be included in a list of warning signals for suicide. The inadequacy feelings that lead young persons to use drugs or alcohol are the same feelings that lead young persons to be suicidal. Substance use reduces teens' ability to think rationally and thus increases the probability of a suicide attempt. It can also lead to risk-taking behavior or miscalculations in attention-getting behavior that can be fatal. The final moments before a suicide attempt are characterized by impaired judgment and decreased contact with reality; substance use only serves to help an adolescent reach that state.

Alcohol in particular is a depressant, and drinking is not a good means for an adolescent to employ to cope with problems. A young adolescent boy graphically described to me how he and his friend got drunk, located a pistol, and began playing Russian roulette. Each boy had pointed the pistol at his head and pulled the trigger once, and then it was my informant's turn again. He pointed the pistol in the air and pulled the trigger, and this time it discharged.

DUNGEONS AND DRAGONS

The relationship of the "Dungeons and Dragons" fantasy game to youth suicide has been questioned. It is estimated that 3–4 million adolescents play the game in the United States. Each player is assigned a character and is encouraged to identify with that character. The game may last for up to several months, with the goal being to accumulate power and to avoid being killed. A recent press release from the National Coalition on Television Violence (1987) emphasized that the game had been a major factor in 26 suicides and 62 murders. The coalition has requested a warning to inform the public about the game. The proponents of the game stress that it promotes cooperation. McDermott (1987) analyzed a number of games and concluded that the link between this game and youth suicide may be overemphasized, although 30 school districts nationwide have banned it. I recommend that school personnel be aware of the game and consider the overall life history and outlook of the students playing it.

RUNAWAYS AND SUICIDE

The personnel of runaway shelters need to be trained in suicide prevention. This need has been recognized in a national movement to train shelter personnel. Brown and Schroff (1986) have found similarities between the profiless of runaways and of suicide attempters. Two other researchers, Engleman (1987) and Fortinsky (1987), addressed the question of how often runaway adolescents are suicidal. They found, respectively, that one in four and one in five runaways in their samples had attempted suicide. Running away from home is a very definite sign that an adolescent is in trouble; school personnel need to recognize this as a warning sign. Shelter personnel and school personnel are both "gatekeepers of the young" who can offer a lifeline.

YOUTHS' CONCEPTS OF DEATH

It is possible to make general assumptions by age group about childrens' and youths' understanding of death; however, young people within an age group will vary in their knowledge and ideas about death (Pfeffer,

1986). Orbach and Glaubman (1979), Davis (1985), and Pfeffer (1986) caution that youngsters often have a mature concept of impersonal death but a rather childish view of their own death. Davis (1985) stresses the limited literature on children's concepts of death, but notes that agreement exists that children do proceed through the following three distinct stages: the preoperational stage, reached at approximately 7 years of age; the concrete operational stage, reached at approximately 10 years of age; and the formal operational stage, reached at approximately 13 years of age.

Children in the preoperational stage can be described as very egocentric; they can perceive themselves as the cause of events, such as the death of another person. They view death as temporary or a state of resting, cannot perceive death as nonexistence, and are unlikely to be motivated to attempt to take their own lives. Children in the concrete operational period view death as real, but external and unlikely to happen to them. Death is seen as happening to the very old. Davis also points out that with increased cognitive abilities in the formal operational period, suicide becomes understandable as a means to an end and is viewed by the adolescent as an option. Death is seen as final, personal, and biological in this stage.

One of the questions that must be addressed is whether or not young children are suicidal. The answer is yes, although it is rare. Children as young as 2 years old have made statements about death and have engaged in risk-taking behavior that is life-threatening. It is difficult to gauge the extent of suicide among very young children as no statistics are kept for children younger than age 5. Among children in the 5–9 age range, a rate of 0.1 per 100,000 has been found (Davis et al., 1988). A general rule is that the younger the child, the less likely it is that the child will have a well-thought-out plan. A young child of elementary age who is suicidal may engage in reckless behavior, such as climbing to high places and running in front of cars.

Pfeffer (1986) has addressed the question of how normal children and suicidal children differ in their ideas about death. Normal children talk about their worries and fantasies about death, but do not have death on their minds as often as suicidal children do.

School personnel need to know how to deal with children who have experienced a death in the family or a death in the school community. A thorough knowledge of the developmental stages of the concept of death is needed, as is a knowledge of the grief process. School personnel must be able to face their own issues having to do with death. They must also help students understand the finality of death.

One of the questions that is difficult to answer concerns how much of our own religious beliefs to share. It is important to allow students their own religious views and to work with these. An adolescent girl with whom I worked provided me with the opportunity to address this issue. The girl's mother and the mother's boyfriend were found dead. The first police report release stated that the mother had killed her boyfriend and then herself; the second report said it was a double murder. There was no conclusive evidence one way or the other. This incident had a profound impact on the 15-year-old girl. She was suicidal and had very detailed plans to end her life. However, her religious beliefs were stopping her from following through on her plans. She believed that her mother had been murdered and was now in heaven. She wanted to rejoin her mother, but her religious belief was that a person who committed suicide would not go to heaven. I emphasized and supported this belief in my efforts to stop her from committing suicide.

TEMPORAL VARIABLES

Is there an "anniversary effect," or some type or a time of year that a suicide attempt is more likely? Baron (1986) cites a study that found that 23% of adolescent suicides died on or near their birthdays. The girlfriend of B (the young man who killed himself as described in Chapter 3) attempted suicide on B's birthday. Another adolescent boy committed suicide a year and a few days after the suicide of his girlfriend. Crisis theory indicates that the anniversary date of a tragedy or a loss is a difficult time for those who are grieving. The mother of an adolescent girl who committed suicide commented, "I think about her the most on the anniversary date, although for a long time I dreaded every Saturday night, as that is when her suicide occurred." School personnel need to be aware that there can be anniversary effects on children.

A widely held belief is that suicide rates are highest during the Thanksgiving-to-Christmas holiday season. There appears to be little evidence to support the theory of increased youth suicide during this holiday season, but there *is* evidence that more young people attempt suicide in the spring (Eyeman, 1987; Porter, 1985; Ruof, Harris, & Robbie, 1987). Phillips and Wills (1987) examined the daily fluctuations of 188,047 U.S. suicides around the national public holidays for a 7-year period from 1973 to 1979. The study found that suicide rates dropped in the days surrounding holidays for every group except white teenagers, who displayed a small, statistically insignificant fluctuation. Phillips and Wills conclude that holidays appear to provide some protection against suicide, but the exact reasons are unknown. A principal recently asked me, "Is there a time of the year that we need to be more alert to teen suicide?" My answer was that we need to be constantly vigilant with our detection efforts.

There is more known about the time of day at which adolescents attempt suicide. Most suicide attempts occur at home between the hours of 3 P.M. and midnight (Indiana State Board of Health, 1985). Porter (1985) reports that 90% of youth suicides occur at home during this time period. This is probably related to the ambivalence that adolescents feel about attempting suicide. They usually attempt suicide at home, when a family member is present who may be able to stop their suicide attempt.

THE IMAGINARY AUDIENCE

The suicidal adolescent often spends considerable time and energy envisioning how other people would react to his or her death. To a certain extent, such imaginings are normal: Everyone has wondered at one time or another what effect his or her death would have on loved ones. How would they react initially? Could they cope and go on with their lives? However, the adolescent who dwells at length on the response of loved ones to his or her death should be considered at high risk for suicide. Davis (1985) suggested that such thoughts may be related to the rise in teen suicide and quoted Elkind who said,

> A common fantasy among suicidal persons is the imagined reactions of an audience. Many suicidal persons see their action as a way of punishing those that they feel rejected them. Such persons take pleasure in imagining the grief and remorse of those they leave behind. These imagined reactions are a powerful motive for carrying out the suicidal idea. (p. 316)

It is important to recognize that a suicidal adolescent's imaginary audience may include not only a parent, boyfriend, or girlfriend, but also the entire student body or a particular class at school. I have had adolescents comment on the amount of attention focused on a teenager who committed suicide. One girl commented, "Everyone is talking about him today, and they all know his name. This school will always remember what he did and may never be the same!" The girl was really impressed by the statement that a boy's suicide had made. More discussion revealed that, yes, she had been thinking about how her friends and the school would react to her own suicide. She did not focus on the reaction of any one person, but instead more on the general impact. I emphasized with this girl the finality of the boy's actions and the reality that life would go on for all concerned; the school would be the same in spite of his action, and he would be thought of less and less as time passed. I asked her whether she had heard of a student named L. She said that she hadn't, and

I stated that she had killed herself 2 years ago. She did not attempt suicide after realizing that L's death had been forgotten.

MANIPULATION AND ATTENTION-GETTING BEHAVIOR

Suicidal ideation and attempts are often attempts to get attention or to manipulate others. A comment made by parents and sometimes school personnel is that a young person is just trying to get attention. Other times, parents may view suicidal behavior as a threat or an attempt to blackmail the parents into giving the child what he or she wants. Berman (1987a) has commented,

> Too often we see angry, conflict-ridden families where suicidal behavior serves as a most powerful weapon in the arsenal of the adolescent intent on manipulating others. Too often, caregivers react pejoratively to adolescents who manipulate. (p. 88)

The question that needs to be asked of parents and school personnel is this: Why is it that this young person feels that he or she can only get attention or change the environment by harming himself or herself? What pattern of life experiences and communication has led to this desperate expression?

A very widely held and very dangerous myth about suicide is the belief that a person who talks about it will not commit suicide. Nothing could be further from the truth, as 80% of suicidal individuals give verbal or behavioral clues. This myth has very great implications as to whether or not to attend to a teenager's suicidal talk. Those who believe this particular myth will not respond at all to the suicidal talk or will respond slowly or in a minimal way. It is vitally important to respond in a very thorough and earnest manner. The young person who does not receive attention when he or she talks about suicide may "up the ante" and take some action in an attempt to get attention, and tragedy may result. For example, an adolescent girl told school personnel of her thoughts of suicide. The counselor followed school procedures and brought the parents to school. The mother stated, "She is just trying to get her way. Every time we take a firm stand and tell her no, she threatens suicide!" The father added, "You people have overreacted in dragging us up here!" It was recommended that counseling be obtained for the girl. The parents voiced their disagreement with the recommendation. Two days later, the girl took pills in an attempt to end her life and had to be rushed to the hospital to have her stomach pumped. A cry for attention? An attempt to manipulate her parents? The answer to both questions is yes, but tragedy could have resulted. Barrett (1985b) suggests that parents "let" themselves be manipulated until professional assistance can be sought, and stresses that when a child is exhibiting suicidal behavior, this is not the time to get tough and crack down on him or her.

DIFFERENCES BETWEEN ADOLESCENTS AND ADULTS WHO ATTEMPT SUICIDE

While both groups have long-standing problems, adolescents who attempt suicide differ from adults who attempt suicide on a number of characteristics. Eyeman (1987) states that suicidal adults have chronic stress problems that wither away their will to live, whereas adolescents' suicide attempts are more likely to result from an acute or transitory reaction to a precipitating event.

Maris (1985) lists a number of ways in which adolescent suicide attempters differ from adult suicide attempters:

1. Adolescents are more impulsive.
2. Adolescent suicide attempts involve more anger, risk taking, and drug abuse.
3. Adolescents are more likely to be influenced by romantic, mystic, and idealistic factors.
4. Adolescents make more nonfatal attempts.
5. Adolescents have more of a family history of divorce and suicide.
6. Adolescents have lower self-esteem and are more influenced by interpersonal relationships.

POETRY, ESSAYS, AND OTHER WRITTEN WORK

Dear Sir

Dear sir
Or father:
Don't blame me for not knowing
What to call you,
For you never called me,
Or wrote me.
Maybe I shouldn't be so harsh,
For you did see me.

Once.
I have the picture
Of you holding me.
It was only for a short time.
And it was the last time.
Why?
From me, my mother receives questions;
From her, I receive no answers.
So now I ask you.
You should see me now,
But some day you will see me,
Or my name,
If only in lights,
And you'll be sorry,
Or maybe even happy
That I don't see you.

The adolescent who wrote this poem committed suicide. School personnel need to pay close attention to suicidal poetry and other written work. In particular, English teachers need to be aware of the facts about youth suicide and alert for indications of it. Every reference to suicide should warn teachers to inquire further and to consider referral through the proper channels at school. Ross (1985a) found 500 poems that contained suicidal thoughts, but were returned to students without comment or follow-up. It is important to look carefully for signs of hopelessness, helplessness, rejection, and loneliness. A student's poem or essay may not contain a direct statement about suicide, but may contain a statement of nonexistence, as in the case of the poem above.

An example of written work that was more specific about suicide was described in a front-page newspaper story in the *Houston Post* on March 21, 1986. The headline read, "Suicide Essay Ends Tragically: Boy Describes Own Death." An 11-year-old boy turned in an essay entitled "Suicide Mistake." The boy committed suicide the evening of the day that he turned in his essay. He employed the method that he had described in his essay.

A study done by Sharlin and Shenhar (1986) compared the poetry of adolescents who committed suicide with that of nonsuicidal adolescents. Differences included a greater use of "loaded words" in the suicide group and a more extreme focus on "Death" and "Bad Situation." Sharlin and Shenhar comment that "adolescent poetry should not be treated with a literary yardstick only, as many teachers do when they receive student poems for reading and evaluation, but should also be studied carefully according to familiarity with the students' biographies and the density of loaded material associated with 'Death' and 'Bad Situation'" (p. 353).

PARENTS AS MODELS

Several researchers have commented that a history of suicide in the family places an adolescent more at risk of trying suicide. Children who survive the suicide of a close family member are believed to be nine times more at risk than other children (Giffin & Felsenthal, 1983). Barrett (1985b) also acknowledges the high correlation that exists between parents who attempt suicide and the attempts of their children.

An example illustrates the importance of parents as models. An adolescent boy was referred to me as being suicidal. The boy and his father were experiencing problems in adjusting to the divorce of his parents. The boy's mother had initiated a divorce and left the adolescent boy to live with his father. He commented, "I had never thought about suicide before, but my dad told me that he was thinking about killing himself and that he had nothing to live for. I was all alone later that night, and I had a few beers and watched the movie *The Deer Hunter*, which showed Russian roulette. I don't know why exactly, but I got out a pistol and pointed it at my head. I almost pulled the trigger; then I threw the gun across the room and went outside."

Pfeffer (1986) comments that "many parents of suicidal children are depressed, suicidal or alcoholic and have poor self-esteem" (p. 132). Friedman, Corn, Jurt, Fibel, Schulick, and Swirsky (1984) found that chronic depression on the part of parents is a strong predictor of adolescent suicide. School personnel need to be aware of the family history and the model of coping utilized by the family. In those cases where a parent has committed suicide, how that loss was communicated to the surviving children is very important, as is the way in which the surviving parent has coped with all the responsibility left to him or her (Klagsburn, 1976). A surviving child may have feelings of guilt, according to Barrett (1985b), and may feel that he or she should have prevented the suicide. It is very interesting to note that three of the four teenagers who committed suicide together in Bergenfield, New Jersey, in March 1987 had parents who had killed themselves (Ryerson, 1987).

SUICIDE METHODS

The *International Classification of Diseases*, ninth edition (World Health Organization, 1977) provides cause-of-death codes for suicide based on mortality files. The CDC (1986) has used this format. Suicide methods are categorized as follows:

- Firearms and explosives
- Hanging, strangulation, and suffocation
- Poisoning by solid or liquid substances
- Poisoning by gases
- Other means

As noted in Chapter 2, the CDC (1986) examined youth suicide in the United States during the period from 1970 to 1980. The data from this report on methods of suicide most frequently employed by males and females are displayed in Tables 4.1 and 4.2, respectively. As the tables indicate, there has been a very definite increase in the number of both male and female suicides utilizing firearms or explosives. Firearms and explosives are now the leading cause of suicide deaths for both males and females. Females previously committed suicide more often through the use of poisoning by solid or liquid substances. Many researchers have called for limiting access to firearms and explosives as one of the most effective ways to reduce youth suicide. Lester (1988) has pointed out the strong correlation between gun ownership and suicide.

THE INFLUENCE OF MUSIC

There has been much discussion about the impact of music on youth suicide. Does music somehow contribute to the suicidal thoughts of a teenager? The idea that music influences suicidal behavior is not a new one. Coleman (1987b) discusses a song entitled "Gloomy Sunday," written in 1933 by a Hungarian composer, which inspired a total of 18 suicides in Hungary.

The song that has received the most publicity in recent years is "Suicide Solution" by Ozzy Osbourne. The song contains the following lyrics:

TABLE 4.1. Most Frequent Methods of Suicide for Males Aged 15-24

Method	1970	1980
Firearms and explosives	51.9%	64.3%
Poisoning by solid or liquid substances	14.1%	5.0%

Note. From *Youth Suicide in the United States, 1970 to 1980* (p. 4) by the Centers for Disease Control, 1986, Atlanta: Author.

TABLE 4.2. Most Frequent Methods of Suicide for Females Aged 15–24

Method	1970	1980
Firearms and explosives	32.3%	52.5%
Poisoning by solid or liquid substances	42.4%	20.0%

Note. From *Youth Suicide in the United States, 1970 to 1980* (p. 4) by the Centers for Disease Control, 1986, Atlanta: Author.

> Breaking laws, locking doors, but there is no one at home.
> Make your bed, rest your head, but you lie there and moan.
> Where to hide? Suicide is the only way out.
> Don't you know what it is really about?

The song has been linked to the suicide of a California teenager. The teenager was reported by Coleman (1987b) to have listened to the song for a period of 5 hours before shooting himself. The parents of the adolescent boy filed suit. Scobie (1986) reported that the suit filed against Osbourne and CBS Records charged that the music encouraged the boy to take his life. Osbourne responded by defending the song as opposing suicide, alcohol, and drugs. Coleman (1987b) summarized the arguments for both attorneys in the case. The attorney for the parents of the deceased argued that Osbourne knew that the song would promote suicide in a violent, morbid, and inflammatory manner. Osbourne's attorney viewed the lawsuit as an assault on artistic freedom, and cited the protection of the First Amendment. A parallel was drawn indicating that Shakespeare contributed to teen suicide by writing *Romeo and Juliet*.

The case was dismissed on August 7, 1986; the presiding judge ruled that the parents' attorney failed to show why the song was not exempt from the First Amendment. The judge stated that "Trash can be given First Amendment protection, too" (quoted in Coleman, 1987b, p. 105).

Coleman (1987b) also reported that a second civil lawsuit was filed in December 1986 against the rock group Judas Priest and CBS Records, after the suicides of two teenage boys in Nevada who spent 6 hours listening to the band's album. The attorney for the parents of one of the deceased boys stated that the lyrics and the intonations of the music "mesmerized" the boy into believing that death was the answer. As of this writing, a trial is expected in late 1988. The argument that the boy was "mesmerized" reminds me of several teenagers' comments on hidden messages contained on records. A number of students have insisted that certain songs played backward encourage suicide. There is no doubt that some teenagers are susceptible to musical references to suicide. The idolization of rock musicians is also a factor. Coleman (1987b) notes that over the last two decades a number of rock stars have committed suicide; the influence of their deaths on young people is believed to be significant, although it is difficult to measure.

A recent movement by a national parent organization, the Parents' Music Resource Center, has attempted to require record companies to publish the lyrics to songs on the outside of album covers so that the lyrics can be read before the albums are purchased. The emphasis is not on censorship, but on informing the consumer. Phyllis Schafly (1985), the President of the Eagle Forum, has commented,

> If you listen to today's rock music, the big question really is, why do we have so few teenage suicides? Rock music lyrics are filled with talk of suicide, death, depression, loneliness, sex and drugs. It's pretty clear that anyone who cares about preventing teen suicide must, first of all, address the problem of rock music. (p. 269)

Barrett (1985b) has summarized the debate about the influence of rock music on youth suicide. The question is whether the music *causes* the suicidal and hopeless feelings, or whether the music simply reflects societal unrest and feelings that are already present in the adolescent. Barrett concludes that there are elements of truth to both positions, and comments,

> [T]he negative effects of music on a healthy adolescent is [sic] probably minimal since their [sic] world is viewed with greater optimism and hope. However, the influence on depressed adolescents is probably different. Their view of the world as bad and not worth being a part of could certainly be reinforced by music with these themes. (1985b, p. 16)

One of the most positive recent attempts to deal with teen suicide through music is Billy Joel's "You're Only Human (Second Wind)." A portion of the royalties from the song and a matching contribution from CBS Records are donated to the National Committee on Youth Suicide Prevention. The song emphasizes the importance of teenagers' giving themselves a second chance.

Music is very important to young people, and much has been written about the effect that music has on them. As noted above, First Amendment issues have been raised in regard to lyrics that deal with suicide. I agree with Barrett's (1985b) statement that suicidal lyrics will have little impact on a healthy adolescent. Music is a form of expression for young people. However, a teenager who listens to music with repeated references to suicide, or to sadness, loneliness, or the like in general, should be considered at risk.

A distraught father of an adolescent boy who had committed suicide brought me the tape that the young man left behind for his family. The adolescent spent considerable time playing various songs that expressed his thoughts and feelings. He said his goodbyes to all in his family, and he spoke of the pain that he was experiencing. He did not blame anyone, but he did not want to go on and face the rest of his life; he saw no end to his pain and heartache. The many songs he played dealt with themes of sadness, loneliness, and failure, but none contained suicidal lyrics. Listening to this boy's final statement was both enlightening and an emotional ordeal. Where do we start with the censorship of musical lyrics, and where do we stop? These are difficult questions to answer. School personnel should recognize that music may have an impact on a troubled teenager. The music that teenagers listen to tells us a lot about how they view the world.

THE INFLUENCE OF MOTION PICTURES
AND TELEVISION

A number of questions have been raised about the impact of depicting suicide in motion pictures. One researcher (Coleman, 1987b) estimated that the average young person, by the time he or she finishes high school, has been exposed to 800 suicides on film.

One film that has drawn a great deal of attention has been *The Deer Hunter*. The question has been raised as to whether this film has caused an increase in the overall suicide rate, or whether it has simply caused a shift in the method employed to commit suicide. The film depicts Russian roulette. Since its release in 1978, there have been 43 such suicides attributed to this movie worldwide (Radecki, 1986).

There are many unanswered questions about the impact of such movies on teenagers. It seems clear that an unhappy, lonely teen who has thought of suicide could be affected by watching a movie depicting suicide. I hope that the producers of such films will begin to exercise some caution. The National Coalition of Television Violence has on several occasions requested that *The Deer Hunter* not be shown by television stations.

Many questions have also been raised about the impact of made-for-television movies that deal with teenage suicide, as well as television news coverage of teen suicide. A heated discussion of these questions took place at the convention of the AAS in May 1987. Several studies have addressed these questions, and considerable debate about the pros and cons of media coverage has taken place.

One concept that needs to be introduced is "the Werther effect." Coleman (1987b) describes the Werther effect as having originated in 1774. In that year, the poet and novelist Johann Wolfgang von Goethe published a book entitled *The Sorrows of Young Werther,* in which the title character commits suicide. A series of suicides occurred in Europe after the publication of *Werther,* and the book was banned in some countries. This imitation effect has implications for all entertainment media, including television, music, books, and motion pictures. David Phillips, a sociologist from the University of California at San Diego, has been the most prominent researcher in this area over the last decade and has conducted a series of research studies to attempt to answer the question of whether or not there is a link between media coverage and suicide. Phillips's research has attracted much attention.

Made-for-television movies dealing with teen suicide became prominent during the 1984–1985 school year. Four such movies were shown by the major networks between October 1984 and February 1985. One of the movies, *Silence of the Heart,* was broadcast on CBS on October 30, 1984. Comments concerning this film by the executive vice-president of CBS, Thomas Leahy, are very informative. Leahy (1985) reported that the film was the most watched program that evening, with a 35% audience share. He gave a number of reasons as to why the film was shown; among them were the need to provide programming that reflected audience concerns and real life. Leahy cited numerous examples of how suicidal teens sought help as a result of the broadcast, and noted that two important messages followed the broadcast. The first was a select bibliography that was prepared by the Library of Congress; the second was a 30-second appeal by Mariette Hartley, who starred in the film, for work on youth suicide prevention. Many local affiliates also provided local resource announcements, such as crisis hotline numbers.

Schafly (1985) criticized a made-for-television movie entitled *Surviving,* shown by ABC on February 10, 1985. This movie depicted two teenagers who died from carbon monoxide poisoning. Unlike *Silence of the Heart,* this movie showed not only the effect the suicides had on the teens' families, but the actual suicides.

Several researchers have attempted to assess what impact made-for-television movies and news coverage have on youth suicide rates. Phillips and Carstensen (1986) examined over 12,000 teen suicides that occurred in the United States from 1973 to 1979. They concluded that youth suicide increased significantly after broadcasts on the subject, and raised the possibility that media coverage may trigger teen suicide. Gould and Shaffer (1986) studied the effects of made-for-television movies on teen suicide in the New York area. They recorded youth suicide attempts and completions during a 25-week observation period from October 1984 to February 1985, during which time four television movies on the subject were shown, and concluded that there was a statistically significant increase; these authors, too, raised the possibility that such movies were somehow triggering teen suicide. They were not sure whether it was the story line, the characters, or the educational material presented that caused the increase, but stressed the need to find out why the increase occurred. Coleman (1987b) cites the research of Alan Berman of American University, who studied the effect of the movie *Surviving*. Data were collected from nine metropolitan areas, and no significant increases in teen suicide were found. However, Coleman notes that several suicides appeared to imitate the methods shown in the movie.

These studies have been challenged by the television networks. Bishop (1986) reported that the television networks found methodological flaws in the research and stressed the large numbers of teens who sought help as the result of watching these broadcasts. The networks also cited professional support for these broadcasts; in addition, professional advisors were used, and educational and preventive materials were provided to affiliate stations.

The media have been faced with some very difficult decisions with regard to suicide. Television networks have also had to address the question of whether or not to show an actual suicide on the news. In January 1987, the state treasurer of Pennsylvania shot himself during a press conference. Several stations showed the suicide in full with a warning to viewers ahead of time, while others chose not to show it.

There has been considerable debate about what role the media should play in reporting teen suicides on the news, and what type of made-for-television movies (if any) should be made on the subject. One concern that I have about television movies on the subject is that the suicidal teens appear to have too much going for them in terms of popularity and attractiveness. The length of a made-for-television movie (1½–2 hours) also does not allow enough time to depict a long-standing pattern of losses, depression, family problems, substance use, and other variables that are known to be factors in teen suicide.

A former president of NBC, Robert Mulholland (1986), has described the concern broadcasters have about this subject. He stresses that limiting public exposure will not stop teen suicide, and adds:

> Experts praise this open communication on a subject that all too long was avoided. To stop this openness now would be taking a giant step backward and doing nothing to get at the causes of teen suicide. The solution is not silence. Broadcasters know that TV can bring the problem into every living room in the country, and it will—responsibly. (p. 10a)

As a counterpoint to Mulholland's remarks, Phillips (1986) has cited research since 1974 linking suicide stories and a rise in deaths just afterwards. Phillips states:

[T]he evidence suggests that suicide stories are not merely precipitating suicides that would have occurred anyway, but are actually creating additional suicides that would not have occurred in the absence of the suicide story. The publicized story seems to be a natural advertisement for one way to cope with life's problems. (p. 10a)

Phillips and Carstensen (1988) have also indicated that news coverage of suicide may affect teenagers more strongly and cause more imitation than in any other age group.

Phillips seems very clear in most of his publications about the link between media coverage and suicide. However, his research has received some criticism, and other research in this area seems inconclusive. In addition, Phillips seems to have contradicted himself recently. On September 24, 1987, *USA Today* ran an article entitled "Teen Suicide Isn't Triggered by TV Movies." The article quoted Phillips as saying, "There's no evidence whatsoever that suicides go up after these programs" (Painter, 1987, p. 1a). Phillips was reported to have found slight *drops* in teen suicide in California and Pennsylvania after three movies were shown in 1984–1985. The article mentioned that this report was welcomed by the Youth Suicide National Center, as earlier studies had caused schools not to show educational films about suicide. I cannot, at this writing, explain the change in the opinion of David Phillips. It appears that his latest position is that made-for-television movies do not cause an increase, but that news coverage does. Shaffer (1988) has surveyed the research in this area and concludes that the news coverage research is consistent, whereas the studies of fictionalized representations of suicide are inconclusive.

I have been concerned that the media link research has been misinterpreted by school personnel. I feel that more, not less, information is needed to prevent suicide. I am in favor of television coverage through carefully screened and prepared fictional and nonfictional stories. I cannot see the value of showing an actual suicide on television, but I can see the value of covering the warning signs and stating where help is available. One of the most powerful aspects of television movies on the subject can be the modeling of intervention by friends. I am in favor of movies that depict suicidal teens being identified and supported by others.

SUMMARY

Many forces and factors affect teen suicide. The search for causation is an elusive one; as many as 28 different factors may play a role (Seibel & Murray, 1988). Much emphasis is placed on family dynamics and family history with regard to coping and modeling. No one type of adolescent is at greater risk for suicide than any other, nor does depression account for all youth suicide. There is growing recognition that conduct problems, impulsivity, substance use, and the availability of firearms are all factors. Teenagers are probably more affected by media coverage of suicide than other age groups; they also may be affected by mystic, romantic, and glorified treatment of suicide in the literature and movies. Teenage suicide is most often a cry for help or an attempt to manipulate others. A precipitating event usually precedes the suicide attempt of an adolescent. Runaway behavior may be a sign that an adolescent is thinking of suicide. The games that adolescents play, the music that they listen to, and the poetry and essays that they write may all be warning signs. School personnel need to keep abreast of the latest trends and research on youth suicide.

5

The School's Role in Prevention and Intervention

A SUCCESSFUL INTERVENTION

Many children and adolescents have been helped by suicide prevention efforts. It is often difficult to measure those efforts that have a positive outcome. Suicide prevention also does not receive the publicity that suicide postvention receives. The following case example is a success story that shows how the school team and prevention efforts can save a life.

R was a new 16-year-old student at a large high school. He had recently come to live with his father. His mother and father had divorced when he was 6 years old; R's mother had remarried when he was 8, and he had adjusted pretty well to the new marriage. R liked his stepfather and continued to visit his father on a regular basis. R had his ups and down, but basically coped well and made satisfactory progress in school. As a teen, he did some experimenting with drugs, but was in a stable peer group.

R's mother divorced his stepfather the summer before his junior year. R took this divorce hard and was angry at his mother; he missed his stepfather, who had moved out of state. R decided to move across town to live with his father. He enrolled as a junior in a large high school (2,500 students), where he did not know many people and made friends very slowly. He kept to himself and didn't interact much with his father. His father worked long hours and spent most of his time with his girlfriend; he provided a car and money for R, but was not emotionally very available. R heard nothing from his stepfather and rarely called or visited his mother. At school, his grades started out as satisfactory, but slowly began to decline. He got an evening job for something to do, but found the job and the evening work hours tiring. R began to buy drugs with the money that he earned.

Eventually, R met a girl named G; he liked her immediately, and they began to date. R had no other close friends and concentrated exclusively on his relationship with G. Things went well at first, but then G indicated that R was too demanding and expressed an interest in seeing other people. He remembered her exact words: "I like you, and we will remain friends, but I need space. You need other friends, not just me. Let's not see each other for a while." R knew that he shouldn't pressure G, but he couldn't help it. She was important to him, and she was all that he had; he had no one else he could really talk to. For the next 2 weeks she seemed to avoid him. R stopped going to classes regularly, and when he did go he couldn't concentrate. He began using more drugs. His work performance went down, and when he skipped work to get high he got fired. When his report card came out, he had failed three of six courses. He decided not to show his grades to anyone. He began thinking of suicide; after all, what did he have to live for?

One Sunday night when his father was out late, R got drunk and decided to poison himself. He found a bottle of aspirin and took all the pills that were in it; he gulped them down with whiskey and fell asleep in his room. The next thing he knew, his father was waking him up. He felt awful and threw up a couple of times. He told his father that he was sick, but stumbled off to school. His father later reported that he thought R had a virus (one that the father had previously had). His father had noticed some changes in R's sleeping and eating patterns, as well as the fact that R was keeping to himself, but he thought that it was all just part of adjustment to the new school. R went to school but sat out in the parking lot. He then decided to get some beer; he went to a store, and then returned to the parking lot and thought again about suicide. He went in to one class and saw G in the hall. When she looked at him, he gave her a funny smile and walked on to class. He sat in class, not hearing the teacher at all as he thought of suicide. It would end his pain when nothing else would. He decided to write a goodbye note to G: "I tried last night with pills to end it all and it didn't work. The next time I'll do it right. Remember me and don't judge me." He left the note in his locker. She had the combination and would find it someday. R left school with a plan to go home and get his gun. He wouldn't survive this time. He would ride around with the gun, have a few more beers, and end it all.

G later reported that she had been worried about R ever since she had asked for space. He just didn't seem the same. He wasn't in school much of the time, and when he was, he just seemed different; he had his head down and didn't seem to be taking care of himself. She had heard that he was using drugs daily and had been seen driving recklessly. That Monday afternoon, he had given her such a strange look that she had a bad feeling about it and decided to go to his locker. She had been to a presentation in health class on adolescent suicide, which covered depression and the warning signs of suicide. She knew R was in trouble, but she still couldn't believe what she found. G did not hesitate: She read the note and ran to the school counselor's office. The door was closed, but G knocked and interrupted the counselor and another student. The counselor saw the panic on her face and took definite action. They both went to the assistant principal, who decided that the first step was to locate R.

R was nowhere to be found. The assistant principal, the counselor, and G decided to go to his house; a second assistant principal was told to call his father. They drove to his house, but he was not there. They decided to call the school to see whether he had been located. As they drove to a pay phone, R passed them in his car on his way home. R pulled into his driveway and was immediately surrounded by the assistant principal, the counselor, and his friend, G. He started to drive off, but the assistant principal said firmly and gently, "We're here to help you. Let's all go in the house and talk." They went in the house and called R's father, who came home immediately. I was also called, and I talked with the father. He agreed to my very firm directives to stay with R all evening and to remove all lethal weapons from the home. We made an appointment for the first thing the next morning.

My interview with R and his father resulted in a referral to an outside mental health professional, who treated R on an outpatient basis initially and then hospitalized him. R has not attempted suicide again. The quick actions of G, the counselor, and the assistant principal probably saved a life. I sent each of them a memorandum complimenting them on their actions, and sent a copy of the memorandum to the principal of the high school.

OVERVIEW OF THE SCHOOL'S ROLE

This example of a successful intervention illustrates how important it is for schools to have a suicide intervention program. Most school districts do not have such a program, for a variety of reasons. One of the most significant reasons is that school personnel are usually not exposed to suicide prevention as part of their training, regardless of whether they are administrators, teachers, counselors, or school psychologists. Harris and Crawford (1987) vividly describe the lack of preparedness and planning in this area in Texas public schools.

This lack of training, coupled with denial about the existence of the problem, has resulted in schools' being slow to develop procedures and direct resources to work on this problem. The OIG (1986) found that responses to proposals to develop suicide intervention programs for teens ranged from fear, denial, and resistance to widespread support. The OIG's report stressed the need for staff training, a student curriculum, and defined referral procedures that are clearly understood and consistently followed. Among administrators and school board members who expressed denial, resistance, or fear, one of the major concerns was that efforts to work on the problem would make it worse. I encountered a memorable denial reaction at an in-service training session I conducted on this topic for all administrators and counselors of a school district of approximately 14,000 students. At the break, one of the principals let me know that he did not think youth suicide was a problem in his community. I asked whether there had been a suicide, and he said no. He implied that my comments and encouragement to develop policies and procedures were not needed. Later checking revealed that two teens had committed suicide in this community in recent years. The administrator did not know the incidence in his own community.

One of the first suicide prevention programs in the schools was begun by Charlotte Ross in San Mateo, California, in 1974. The program was developed in response to a total of 11 suicides in the school system (Colt, 1984). This program has served as a model for others to follow. Ross (1985a) notes that educators care and want to reduce youth suicide, but fear and ignorance hold them back. They have their own feelings of ambivalence and denial and are worried about blame. Ross emphasizes that programs in the schools are workable and feasible. Such programs can help young people understand depression and can mobilize resources in the community to work on this problem.

The program begun by Ross in San Mateo emphasizes two key points. First, it teaches school personnel that they can be the "gatekeepers" of the young and can detect suicidal students. Second, the program emphasizes the importance of talking about suicide in our society and encourages suicidal youths to get help. Ross stresses that the rule of silence, which discourages discussion of suicide, prevents many young people from getting the assistance that they need. Ross emphasizes the need for clearly defined procedures to prevent suicide, in which the roles of various school personnel are made explicit. Ross acknowledges that assuming the responsibility of being a "gatekeeper" is scary for school personnel; they need encouragement, reminders, and refresher in-service sessions to translate knowledge about prevention into action. Ross stresses that when teachers talk about suicide, they do not cause students to become suicidal. She points out the need to involve both teacher organizations and parent organizations in suicide prevention. The program that Ross has developed does emphasize curriculum presentations for students on this topic, and more information about these presentations is given in Chapter 10. A final comment from Ross is very straightforward: "The use of educational programs as an effective approach to the reduction of suicidal death is well established in the field of suicidology" (1985a, p. 151).

Thomas Barrett developed and directed the Cherry Creek School's (Colorado) suicide prevention project, which was federally funded and began in 1980. He has written extensively about youth suicide prevention. Barrett (1985b), in addressing the question of who are the caregivers, has stated, "Traditionally, the assumption has been made that mental health professionals were the only ones who could recognize the symptoms of self-destructive behavior. The problem is that such professionals are too few and too inaccessible" (p. 41). Barrett also argues that it is incorrect to assume that only individuals with professional degrees should deal with suicidal youths. I readily agree with this point; I have seen school bus drivers, for example, make a difference and take action to prevent a suicide. Suicide prevention information is now provided to all bus drivers in my school district. Barrett's key points are that all school personnel who interact with students on a daily basis need skills in dealing with suicide, and that all school personnel have a role to play.

Barrett has also noted that some mental health professionals do not support an active prevention effort in the schools; the substance of their argument, as noted earlier, is that talking about the problem somehow causes it. Barrett (1985a) provided a rebuttal to comments of this type made by psychiatrist Derek Miller at an AAS convention. Miller stated, "We spent a fair amount of time discussing what I understand is a strange aberration in this state, the concept of educating about suicide in the schools which struck me as a most terrifying concept" (quoted in Colt, 1984, p. 3). Barrett cited others who have expressed similar views and have used the argument that talking about the drug problem in the schools has resulted in the problem's becoming worse. Barrett's reaction to Miller's comments was this: "His comments did not trouble me as much as the silence that followed it. Miller was challenging what seems to the major thrust of the adolescent suicide movement—education in the schools, and his challenge went unmet" (1985a, p. 3).

Barrett (1985b) has addressed several other major points about the role of the schools and emphasizes that those in the schools should have no philosophical problem with intervening to stop the suicide of a young person. Critical factors in establishing a program are establishing a need, fostering support from parents and the community in general, and getting a commitment from the school system. Barrett stresses the importance of the school program's being coordinated with state and community agencies. The Cherry Creek curriculum emphasizes basic information on suicide prevention, intervention strategies, alternatives to suicide, and community resources. Discussion pamphlets are provided to students and parents. Barrett (1985a) has found that students who are taught this information report increased knowledge of the warning signs and more confidence in their ability to help a suicidal friend in the future. The role of peers in this model is limited to identification, referral, and support of a friend, and does not include peers in a counseling role. An emphasis is also placed on welcome and orientation for new students in the school district (Barrett, 1985b). Berkovitz (1985) has emphasized the importance of the school's having an overall atmosphere of positive mental health and optimal psychological and counseling services.

Garfinkel (1986), in reviewing a number of existing school-based suicide prevention programs, has made a number of recommendations as to what a comprehensive program should contain. Garfinkel stresses that a number of school programs are not comprehensive enough. The components recommended by Garfinkel are as follows:

1. Early identification and screening to enable school personnel to detect adolescents at risk and to understand the major stressors that adolescents face and the behavioral symptoms they exhibit.
2. A comprehensive evaluation of the suicidal youth, including a structured psychiatric interview, self- and clinician ratings, and psychometric testing.
3. Crisis intervention and case management procedures to alleviate the stress the adolescent is experiencing and set a course of action to provide needed assistance.
4. Postvention programs to assist those who survive a suicide.
5. Education programs for school personnel, students, parents, and the community, emphasizing coping skills, prevention, intervention, and postvention.
6. Monitoring and follow-up of those youths who are at risk and those most affected by a suicide.
7. Community linkage and networking with other schools, community agencies, media personnel, and community organizations.
8. Research concerning causation and epidemiology.
9. Advocacy to work on youth suicide prevention, with the school system becoming a resource for the community to work on this problem.

Garfinkel (1986) has commented,

The most important function of all is for the suicidal student to have an advocate readily available eight hours, five days per week to be knowledgeable about the thoughts and feelings the student is experiencing, to more effectively interpret the individual's behavior towards others and to accomplish these tasks in an empathic fashion to the students. It is estimated [that] between 3–6% of all high school students will require the direct services of a suicide prevention team. Not only . . . at risk students, but all students, teachers, and members of the community will benefit from the diverse activities of this team. (p. 12)

Johnson and Maile (1987) have also discussed the role of school in suicide prevention. They recommend that school personnel be trained to be alert for warning signs, stress the importance of replacing the many myths held about suicide with factual information, and emphasize the difference that an alert and knowledgeable school staff member can make in saving a life. The school system can do much to promote mental health for students and has a moral responsibility to do so. Johnson and Maile believe that the reluctance of schools to work on the problem is due to ambivalent feelings, uncertainty about the schools' responsibility, denial about the problem, and the desire not to be manipulated by the suicidal gestures of students.

I view the role of the school as very straightforward, and I devote the rest of this chapter to outlining it and describing the roles that various school personnel should play in addressing this problem. I recommend that each school have in place a basic suicide intervention program, regardless of size; however, the size of a school and whether it is located in an urban, a suburban, or a rural area are important factors. Additional components need to be added in school districts that are urban or suburban. The most comprehensive intervention efforts are in place in those schools that have experienced multiple suicides (OIG, 1986). Other questions that arise have to do with what a suicide prevention program should consist of and who should carry it out. Should the program be ongoing, and should the program be school- or community-based?

As I see it, the role of the school should be as follows:

1. To detect suicidal students.
2. To assess the severity level of their suicidal thoughts and/or actions.
3. To notify parents.
4. To secure needed supervision and services for the students.

These four points seem very simple to describe, but can be very complicated to put in place. They should be at the core of any school program, regardless of the size of the school, and should be clearly outlined in written school policy. One of the benefits of having a written policy is to limit the responsibility of the school.

I am supportive of all the components mentioned by Ross (1985a), Barrett (1985b), and Garfinkel (1986). I also support curriculum programs, media guidelines, and postvention procedures, and have devoted a chapter of this book to each. However, I am also a realist. A giant first step would be to implement the four basic points listed previously. I have given presentations to superintendents on several occasions, and they are reluctant to begin a comprehensive suicide intervention program. Few, if any, school administrators are ready to implement all nine points recommended by Garfinkel (1986) at once. The suicide intervention program that I have directed has evolved and gotten more comprehensive over the years with constant review.

Capuzzi (1987) stresses what I believe is a key point—that we must train the school faculty first before we approach students, give them information about suicide, and encourage them to open up about their suicidal thoughts. Teachers must know what to do and how to refer students, and the school counselor must know how to assess the severity of a student's symptoms, notify parents, and secure services for the student.

GAINING ADMINISTRATIVE SUPPORT

The key to whether a suicide intervention program is implemented in a school is whether the top administrators support the program. I have already described at some length the reluctance of administrators to devote resources to this problem. How can we avoid having to experience one or more suicides before a program is authorized? I have talked with numerous school personnel who have tried to establish an intervention program but have not received any encouragement, or, in some cases, have been told that a program is not needed.

Lennox (1987) has emphasized the importance of a clear, step-by-step policy. Boggs (1987) has also emphasized the importance of a comprehensive policy to guide the actions of a school, and has pointed out that schools can actually contribute to the problem of youth suicide if they minimize and ignore it. Vidal (1986) stresses that private mental health professionals are ready and willing to assist the schools at little or no cost if the schools would let them. Shipman (1987) has emphasized the prevalence of the problem and stated that schools can and must have formalized programs. Such programs need administrative and school board support, with the acknowledgment that doing something places the school in less jeopardy than doing nothing. Johnson and Maile (1987) note that administrators set the tone for an individual school and the system as a whole, and are the key to prevention efforts; these authors comment, "Where the school is unprepared or reluctant to become in-

volved, it is apparent to us that the tragedy is markedly compounded"
(p. vii).

Written procedures are essential, but they need not all be the same.
Each school system should examine the problem in its community and
develop a program that meets its needs and utilizes its resources. The
most controversial question is whether or not to present information
about suicide prevention to students. This does not have to be the first
thing that is done, and this debate should not interfere with establishing
system guidelines to detect and assist suicidal students. I recommend that
school personnel pursue the following strategies in a persistent and
professional manner to gain administrative support:

1. Job descriptions for school psychologists, counselors, and social
workers should include suicide intervention.

2. The importance of having in place written procedures prior to the
crisis, to guide everyone and to limit the responsibility of the school,
must be emphasized. The existence of such procedures will be invaluable
in answering to the public and the media, should a suicide occur.

3. Administrators should be provided with information about the
incidence at the national, state, and local level. Copies of magazine or
newspaper articles will highlight the need and emphasize that no school
is immune. Several administrative journals have contained excellent articles on this subject written by administrators.

4. School personnel should obtain samples of guidelines and procedures used by other school districts and use these in making written
recommendations for their district.

5. Personnel should have the proper information and training in this
area to give their recommendations more credibility.

6. Personnel should gather data about the number of attempts and
completed suicides in the school district over a several-year period.

7. When school personnel work with a suicidal youth, they should
make sure that administrators are notified.

8. Examples should be provided of how the schools have intervened
to assist a suicidal youth and save a life.

9. Personnel may suggest that the superintendent ask the school
district's attorney for his or her opinion.

10. Administrators should be provided with information about the
legislation requiring programs in some states.

My experience has been that secondary school counselors, psychologists, and nurses are dealing with suicidal youths on a regular basis, and
they are desperate for support and guidance from the administration.
Such support in writing does much to alleviate their fears and encourage

all school personnel to assist suicidal youths. It is also important, after administrative support is obtained, to give the superintendent and principals feedback on intervention efforts. I was once in the hallway of a high school after a suicide, talking to the principal, when the superintendent walked up and inquired how the students were coping. The principal responded, "They are coping as well as can be expected, thanks to the invaluable assistance of the psychology department!"

A MODEL OF SUICIDE INTERVENTION

Every school needs a model to guide its efforts to work on the problem of youth suicide. The work of Caplan (1964) in crisis intervention provides a theoretical basis for developing a suicide intervention program. According to Caplan, there are three distinct levels of intervention when a crisis occurs: primary prevention, secondary intervention, and tertiary intervention. Most school personnel think only of what they do in the immediate aftermath of a crisis, and not about what could have been done to prevent the crisis or what long-term follow-up and assistance students and faculty will need. Primary prevention consists of what can be done to stop a crisis from happening through eliminating hazards or modifying the situation. Secondary intervention involves providing immediate assistance to an individual or group in handling a crisis, with the purpose of minimizing the effects of the crisis. Tertiary intervention involves providing long-term assistance to those affected by a crisis; the goal is to assist the individual or group to resume precrisis functioning without any lasting debilitating effects. The three levels of intervention are sometimes described as prevention, intervention, and postvention, respectively.

Johnson and Maile (1987) have provided a very thorough discussion of crisis intervention principles with regard to suicide intervention. They make the following points: In primary prevention, students are taught skills to manage situations, and knowledge is provided to the school community about intervening to assist suicidal students. In secondary intervention, help is provided to an individual or group because of a suicidal crisis. In tertiary intervention, help is given to an individual or group if problems persist after the immediate crisis has been resolved.

This theoretical model is not one with which school administrators are familiar, but I have found that they grasp it quickly and that they particularly like the emphasis on preventing a suicidal crisis from occurring. Table 5.1 summarizes the suicide intervention activities that comprise the program in the Cypress–Fairbanks (Texas) Independent School District.

TABLE 5.1. Levels of Suicide Intervention and Specific Activities

Primary prevention
- Annual in-service training session for all secondary school faculty, emphasizing the warning signs and referral procedures, with handout.
- Annual training provided to counselors and nurses.
- Training provided to teachers in subjects such as health, psychology, and sociology.
- Curriculum presentations to students in selected subjects.
- Presentations to student groups.
- Community- and school-based presentations for parents emphasizing mental health and suicide prevention.
- Articles written on suicide prevention published in local newspapers and district newsletters, sent to each parent.
- Group counseling provided weekly to approximately 350 "at-risk" secondary students.
- Establishment of welcoming clubs and activities to help new students.
- Various school activities to boost student morale and promote a positive and drug-free school.
- Establishment of teen helpline programs.

Secondary intervention
- Provision of immediate support to a suicidal student.
- Assessment of the severity level of the student's suicidal thoughts or actions.
- Notification of the parents of a suicidal student.
- Securing of needed services for the suicidal students, with or without parental support.
- Activities to assist faculty and students through the grieving process immediately following a suicide, and to minimize the contagion effects of the suicide.
- Identification of those students most affected by the suicide, and provision of assistance.
- Suggestion of appropriate memorials to the deceased.
- Responses to media attention that encourage downplaying the suicide method employed and instead publicize where to get help.
- Contact with the parents of the student who committed suicide, to offer sympathy, care for surviving siblings, and coordination of services between the school and family.

Tertiary intervention (postvention)
- Long-term follow-up of those who have been affected by the suicide of a friend or relative.
- Awareness of anniversary dates of losses and the birthdays of significant others who have committed suicide, and provision of support to those who need it at those difficult times.

Much has been written about the role of the school. In regard to primary prevention, there has been a debate about whether or not a distinction should be made between activities aimed at the entire student body and early identification of suicidal youths (Felner, 1987). Much time could be spent in detailing the hundreds of activities that could be done to promote mental health and problem-solving skills for young people. These activities are very important, but it is not necessary to outline them all, nor could any one person do so. One primary prevention effort that deserves mentioning is the organization called Students Against Suicide, which was created by teenagers and has stopping teenage suicide as its goal. Hardy (1985) states that the group promotes learning the warning signs and knowing what to do to help a suicidal friend. Commitment to life is emphasized, and a variety of fund-raising and speaking projects are carried out. The Youth Suicide National Center can provide more information about this group (see Chapter 12 for the center's addresses).

The most salient point is that a suicide intervention program should be comprehensive and involve several different levels of intervention. The four basic aspects of the school's role, as outlined earlier in this chapter— that is, detection, assessment, notification of parents, and securing of appropriate services for suicidal students—fit well into Caplan's (1964) model. However, the role of the school should not be interpreted to include diagnosis and treatment, and school resources must be coordinated to ensure consistent, comprehensive intervention (Shipman, 1987). Finally, key points in any crisis program include initial and continuing planning and evaluation of the program.

GETTING THE PROGRAM UNDERWAY

Once administrative support has been secured and a model has been used to outline the levels of intervention, many questions remain. What should the school system do first? As I see it, procedures should be written to outline the training efforts and clarify who is going to do what to assist suicidal youths and prevent suicides. I agree with Capuzzi (1987) that the faculty must be trained first. Some school districts have used a required in-service training session for all teachers; this is usually scheduled in late summer before school begins. Such sessions reach all teachers, but usually in a large-group format that prohibits discussion. Some school districts, including the one that I work for, have approached the problem differently. We elected to train nurses and counselors first and emphasized not only the warning signs, but also assessment, notification, and obtaining services. We chose to do so because nurses and counselors are the school personnel teachers most often go to for help. Next, information was presented to principals. Presentations to teachers followed in a small-group format that took over a year to reach all teachers. It took another year to reach other personnel, such as aides and bus drivers.

Another point to be kept in mind in regard to getting a program underway is that someone must be assigned the responsibility to coordinate the program and continually evaluate and update it. As the director of psychological services for the Cypress–Fairbanks School District, I volunteered to fulfill that role, and I annually make a report to the superintendent. If responsibility is not clarified, then programs either do not get off the ground or become dormant. It can often be unclear whose job it is to do what in the schools. There are also many time constraints placed on school personnel. The Dallas Independent School District dealt with this problem in a very creative and effective way. The school board authorized the creation of three new psychology positions to deal only with crisis intervention; these psychologists have no other duties. According to Smith (1987), several parents who had survived the suicide of a child appeared before the Dallas school board and urged that more be done to prevent youth suicide. The Dallas program emphasizes extensive training for school counselors. A primary caregiver is selected and trained on every campus, with the three crisis psychologists available to provide assistance.

I believe that each school system should make its own decisions about how to train school personnel and who is going to provide such training. A small rural school district may need to bring in an outside consultant to train the faculty. A large school district may prefer to send its own psychological staff to a workshop and then have the staff members train the district faculty. A recommendation that such training should be voluntary for school staff, because of how much anxiety the topic invokes, has been made by Heiman, Jones, Lamb, Dunne-Maxim, and Sutton (1985). I acknowledge the anxiety, but feel that school personnel need the training and will not be resistant to it if approached properly. Information about suicide prevention needs to be presented to all who work in the schools, with periodic reviews and reminders.

DEVELOPING THE IN-SERVICE TRAINING SESSION FOR SCHOOL PERSONNEL

Goals

A very basic question is what the goals for an in-service training session should be. I think the goals should be the following:

1. To give school personnel knowledge about the warning signs of suicide.
2. To eliminate the misperceptions about suicide.
3. To provide accurate information about the incidence of youth suicide and causation factors.
4. To clarify the school system's procedures.
5. To empower personnel with the knowledge that they can make a difference and save a life.
6. To clarify their role in suicide intervention.
7. To clarify issues having to do with confidentiality, to emphasize that *school personnel must not keep secrets* about suicidal behavior.
8. To identify community resources.

Johnson and Maile (1987) emphasize building morale and encouraging school staff that they can do something to help. They believe that it is important to emphasize the high incidence of suicide, the need for individual response capabilities, and the effectiveness of school personnel in intervening. The Wisconsin Department of Instruction (1986) gives the following objectives for a faculty in-service session:

1. To sensitize faculty members to the problem and help them understand the stresses that teens face.
2. To promote an understanding of the warning signs.
3. To improve faculty–student communication.
4. To clarify referral procedures.
5. To outline crisis intervention strategies.
6. To identify community resources.

This guide also addresses the moral questions of whether faculty members have a right to intervene to prevent teen suicide and whether it is their responsibility to do so. These questions need to be addressed, and the faculty needs to understand that the answer to both questions is yes. Barrett (1985b) and Heiman et al. (1985) suggest beginning the in-service session by acknowledging that this is a difficult topic to talk about. I have found that when I talk to a group about suicide prevention, someone in the group has usually experienced the loss of a friend or family member through suicide. I acknowledge the suicide of my own father and make myself available to school staff members who wish to talk more privately after the session. I also state that my goal is to give the group members correct information about teenage suicide and what they can do to prevent it.

Preparation, Content, and Method of Presentation

It is essential that the presenter be well prepared. I have found it easier to give presentations on this topic over the years as my knowledge and confidence have grown. I recommend careful preparation and rehearsal. I have found it effective to get the attention of the school personnel by reading them one or two poems written by suicidal youths. I also often give them a test on their information about youth suicide when they enter the room. I hand them the test and have them look over it before I begin my presentation. The information test appears in Appendix B of this book, and the answers appear in Appendix C.

Lennox (1987) recommends that factual information about suicide be presented, including information about incidence, myths, causation, substance use, stress, family dynamics, warning signs, identification of high-risk students, the importance of a prior attempt, and depression. Lennox also points out the importance of clarifying the policies and procedures for the school system. Administrative support should be stressed, and professional issues such as confidentiality, ethics, and responsibility should be clarified. Lennox recommends that school personnel be given examples of how to respond and what to say to a suicidal student. School personnel must also understand the vulnerability of survivors to suicidal thoughts after the suicide of a classmate. Other areas emphasized by Lennox include support for school staff; the fact that it is okay to talk about suicide; the staff's responsibility to help others; and the fact that because of the situational nature of suicide, the intervention of one person can make the difference. Small-group presentations are recommended, with follow-up discussion so that the participants can explore their personal reactions. The presentation should avoid glorifying suicide; if films are used, they should be carefully reviewed. A handout detailing the warning signs and indicating what to do to help a suicidal student should be provided. Some school districts have distributed brochures on suicide prevention.

Barrett (1985b) also recommends small-group presentations, with the emphasis on personal philosophies about suicide, professional issues such as liability and confidentiality, and practical details about what to do to assist suicidal students. Boggs (1987) found that 92% of elementary teachers and 100% of secondary teachers who had been trained in suicide prevention recommended that this information be shared with all teachers. The teachers reported that they increased their knowledge of the symptoms of suicidal behavior, as well as their ability to respond and get help for students. I find it very interesting that teachers want this information but that administrators are reluctant to approve such in-service sessions. Harris and Crawford (1987) found that administrators gave such sessions very low priority unless multiple suicides had occurred.

I have found it not merely helpful but necessary to read a few quotes to address the questions of whether we should talk about suicide. I find the following quote helpful: "You will never give a kid the idea of committing suicide by talking about it. In fact, just knowing someone is available and interested may be the factor that will save his life" (Cantor, 1985, p. 85).

I have had the opportunity to give presentations to numerous school groups. Everyone needs the same basic information. The smaller the group the better; however, sometimes it is necessary to address large groups of school personnel to get this important information to them quickly. The ideal group size is 10–40 people. What length of time is needed to get across this information? I recommend 1–2 hours. A 2-hour session allows time to show an educational film. I have found school staff to be very interested in this information; almost without exception, there has been a teenage suicide previously in the community. Table 5.2 gives a sample outline for a school in-service session.

Warning Signs of Suicide

School personnel need to know and recognize the warning signs of suicide. I use examples of actual verbal statements and behavioral clues given by suicidal teens. Examples of verbal statements are "What would it be like to be shot in the head with a gun?" or "I won't be at the party Saturday; by then I will be in hell!" Behavioral clues may include giving away prized possessions, making out a will, and making a list of loved ones that the teen wants to see one more time. The AAS publication *Suicide & How to Prevent It* (1977) lists the following as warning signs:

- Suicide threats or similar statements
- An attempt at suicide
- Prolonged depression
- Dramatic change of behavior or personality
- Making final arrangements

I point out to school personnel the importance of responding to obvious verbal and behavioral clues of suicidal behavior. I recommend that staff members inquire directly and ask whether students who give such clues are thinking of harming or killing themselves. A staff member needs to give a clear message: "I am here to help you and I care about you." The California State Department of Education (1987) outlines ways in which school personnel can respond to help suicidal students:

TABLE 5.2. Suicide Prevention In-Service Session: Outline

Topic	Approximate time
Poems	3– 5 minutes
Statement of purpose	3– 5 minutes
Clarification of the school's role	5–10 minutes
Incidence figures	5–10 minutes
Facts versus myths	10–15 minutes
Movie	20–30 minutes
Warning signs	5–10 minutes
Confidentiality and other ethical, professional, and liability issues	10–20 minutes
How can school personnel help?	5–15 minutes
Referral procedures	5–10 minutes
A success story	10 minutes
Identification of community resources	5–10 minutes
Legislation	3– 5 minutes
Questions	5–15 minutes
Conclusion—empowerment	3– 5 minutes

1. Listen without making judgments. Be alert to suicidal intent.
2. Don't hesitate to inquire directly about suicide.
3. Be honest and open; encourage discussion and share your feelings.
4. Ask the student questions.
5. Communicate concern and support through reaching out.
6. Offer resources. Be hopeful and positive.
7. Act quickly.

School staff members may be very concerned that they might say the wrong thing. They need to let the basic helping desire that brought them into education in the first place guide their inquiry. They need to act from the heart and show concern, and must not dismiss or minimize the suffering these adolescents are experiencing. They need to reach out and let the adolescents know that they care, rather than preaching to them.

It is helpful to provide the faculty with a scenario such as the following, to help them to be alert to the warning signs and the importance of direct inquiry:

Billy, a 16-year-old student in your class, hasn't seemed the same since his mother died of cancer 3 months ago. His grades have fallen, and he has been moody and irritable in your class. You have noticed that he's not taking as much pride in his appearance. You have heard rumors that he has been using drugs. Today he wrote on the bottom of his homework, "If my

girlfriend ever broke up with me, then I would have nothing to live for."
What should you do?

The faculty should have an opportunity to respond and be guided
through making a direct inquiry into Billy's suicidal thoughts. A key
point is that a teacher will not cause Billy to be suicidal by inquiring
about it. Open-ended questions or reflective statements should be used,
such as the following:

- "You don't seem yourself lately."
- "Your school work has fallen off."
- "Your mother's death has been very hard on you."
- "Your girlfriend is very important to you."

A more direct inquiry about suicidal thoughts should follow:

- "You sound as if you think you have little to live for."
- "Have you thought about giving up?"

It then may be necessary to inquire about suicidal plans or actions:

- "Have you thought about how you would end your life?"

Support can be offered through the following statements:

- "You aren't the first person to feel this way."
- "There is help available to you."

At this point, the teacher needs to follow the referral procedures. Acting
quickly is important; depending on Billy's answers, it may not be advisable to leave him alone. The staff member then needs to refer Billy,
according to the school's referral procedures, to a trained counselor or
school psychologist who will make a thorough assessment of the situation. Sometimes school staff members bring up the fact that they would
be violating the student's confidence. I respond by saying that we cannot
keep secrets about suicidal behavior, and that Billy is probably relieved
that someone now knows how he is feeling and is trying to help. I also
stress that school personnel are wonderful, caring human beings, but
they are not trained to assess the severity level of a student's suicidal
thoughts or actions. They must refer Billy so that he can get help, and so
that the school staff member is not carrying around a tremendous responsibility that could leave him or her open to professional and personal
liability.

The California State Department of Education (1987) lists the following sudden changes in school behavior as possible indications that a student is suicidal:

1. Dramatic changes in attendance.
2. Declining academic performance and failure to complete work.
3. Withdrawal from activities and friends.
4. Frequent talk or writing about death and despair.
5. Mood swings.
6. Dramatic change in appearance or personality.
7. Increased usage of drugs and alcohol.

The Wisconsin Department of Instruction (1986) also addresses the indicators of teen suicide. The department recommends that school personnel look for a cluster of indicators, such as personality changes, increased alcohol or drug usage, eating or sleeping changes, depression, withdrawal from activities and interpersonal relationships, verbal and behavioral clues, and difficulty making even minor decisions. Several behaviors are noted as masking teen depression, and it is recommended that school personnel be alert for truancy, running away, neglecting school work, and violent behavior.

It is often suggested that school personnel look for a certain type of student when trying to detect suicidal behavior. Perfectionists, risk takers, loners, abused and neglected children, students with low self-esteem, depressed students, gays and lesbians, drug users, teenagers in trouble with the law, and learning-disabled students are all mentioned as at risk by the California State Department of Education (1987). My recommendation to school personnel is that they not look for one type of student, but instead recognize that each student is unique and that suicide occurs across all socioeconomic and racial boundaries. It is very important to pay attention to the loss history of a student. Have there been recent losses, disappointments, or humiliations? Has the student ever threatened or attempted suicide previously? Is there a history of suicide in the family? Does the student use alcohol or drugs? Such information is very helpful in identifying teens at risk.

As noted earlier, confidentiality issues must be addressed with the faculty. A teacher at a workshop once asked a question that I find helpful to use in addressing the confidentiality issue: "A boy in my class told me last year about his suicide attempt. He made me promise not to tell anyone, and I haven't. I don't think anyone knows about this but me—certainly not his parents. Did I do the right thing?" I let the group answer this question. The answer that I am looking for is that the teacher did not do the right thing and accepted far too much responsibility. The parents needed to know about this, because the boy might attempt suicide again as a way of dealing with his problems.

Films

I have found it helpful to show a film about teenage suicide at an in-service session. The film can reinforce key points and help to give the school staff members increased confidence that they can prevent a suicide. I use two films the most frequently, although any number of films could suffice. I do recommend that each film be previewed carefully, so that there are no discrepancies between the information in the film and what is being presented in the session.

The first film, *Suicide—The Warning Signs* (Coronet Films, 1984), is 24 minutes long and is distributed by Coronet Films, 420 Academy Drive, Northbrook, IL 60062. The film version costs $525, the video cassette costs $290, and the rental fee is $70. This film does a very thorough job of covering the warning signs and emphasizing that suicide can be prevented. The film contains three vignettes of high-school-age or college-age students. The first shows Greg, who is accident-prone, standing on the roof of his school and threatening to jump. The second vignette shows Carol, who is contemplating suicide. She throws the pills she is thinking of taking into a field, but then searches for them and finds them. She gives her parents numerous verbal and behavioral clues. The third vignette depicts Curtis, who has been depressed over the breakup with his girlfriend and gives away prized possessions. Curtis leaves a note for a friend, who does not hesitate and finds Curtis just as he is getting out a handgun.

This film does an excellent job of presenting the basics about suicide prevention. It does have a somber tone; in addition, Carol follows through on her suicide attempt, and although the outcome is not clear, scenes at the cemetery give the impression that she succeeded. Another possible problem is that the film does show several methods of suicide, which could conceivably result in imitation if the film were to be shown to students. A positive aspect of the film is that two of the three suicidal youths are detected and receive assistance. The film also features several minority characters.

The second film, *Young People in Crisis*, lasts 35 minutes and is a combined film presentation of the National Committee on Youth Suicide Prevention and the AAS (1987). This film can be purchased or rented from Exar Communications, Inc., 267B McClean Avenue, Staten Island, NY 10305. The film version costs $250, the video cassette costs $75, and the rental fee is $35–$50. A discussion guide and 30 take-home booklets are provided. This film is designed to emphasize the warning signs and to convince school personnel and parents that they can help save a life. The film features Dr. Pamela Cantor, a former president of the AAS. Cantor lectures on various important points, and several vignettes depict young people who are suicidal.

This film does not depict a suicide; instead, it emphasizes intervention by friends and school personnel. The film also avoids showing young people with lethal instruments. Methods of suicide and the impact that a suicide has on others are downplayed. There is no glorification or sensational treatment of the subject. The situational nature of suicide and the intervention of others to save a life are emphasized. Cantor (1987) stresses that the film is appropriate for teenagers; in fact, she states that schools are the target audience. This is a film that I recommend highly, and the modest cost for a videocassette makes this a film that every high school should have. One possible criticism of the film is that it has no minority students in it.

Other Considerations

The initial in-service session for all school faculty is the cornerstone to a prevention program. Faculty members need to know what to look for and what to do. They also need an awareness of what happens when they refer a student to the counselor or psychologist. I explain that the counselor or psychologist will assess the severity level of the student's symptoms, notify parents, and work toward securing services for the student. The referring faculty member will be given some feedback and an update on what is being done to assist the student. The school personnel want to make certain that efforts are being made to assist the student. I emphasize that the counselor or psychologist has received special training in working with suicidal students. School personnel also need to know what resources are available in the community, such as crisis hotlines and how they work. Students should not be given the crisis hotline number as an alternative to following school referral procedures; instead, the hotline number should be used in conjunction *with* referral procedures. Each state varies on mandated procedures for dealing with suicidal students, and school faculty need to know the status of legislation in their state. Evaluative information should be gathered concerning whether or not the faculty members' knowledge and confidence in detecting and dealing with suicidal students have increased.

Suicide is a heavy topic, and in sessions that last for more than an hour, some relief is needed. I have a Tom and Jerry cartoon that provides some humor. The cartoon portrays a very sad bird who tries to commit suicide. The bird is prevented from doing so by his friend, Jerry. Jerry snatches him from the jaws of the mean cat, Tom, on several occasions. The cartoon ends very happily when the bird meets a lady bird and they stroll off into the sunset. A cartoon featuring Loopy DeLoop, produced by Hanna-Barbera, has a similar storyline. Audiences love these cartoons, and readily understand both that the intervention of a friend can be powerful and that the nature of suicide is situational. I have several anecdotes that I also tell to provide some humor. It is very important to provide this humor and to close the in-service session with a "success story," such as the one that begins this chapter.

Ross (1985a) stresses the need for follow-up presentations. I have found it helpful to make short annual presentations to review key points and give staff the opportunity to ask questions. The handout entitled "Teenage Suicide Prevention Tips" (Schindler & Poland, 1985), contained in Appendix A of this book, is distributed annually to all secondary school faculty in my district.

ASSESSMENT

It is vitally important that someone in the school system be skilled at assessing the severity level of a suicidal student's symptoms. There are those who would disagree with this notion and recommend that each and every suicidal student be immediately transported to the local mental health center. There are countless reasons why this is not always possible or recommended. Brown and Schroff (1986) emphasize that preliminary assessment can be done by other than mental health professionals— indeed, *must* be done, or valuable time is wasted. This assessment does not take the place of mental health treatment or attempt to solve all the student's problems; instead, it offers support for the student and starts in motion steps to help the student.

The assessment of suicidal risk is very logically done by counselors, school psychologists, social workers, or nurses. Most of the time, this task falls to the school counselor. The responsibility of assessing the suicidal potential of students often causes great anxiety for counselors; this is not a task for which they were prepared in graduate school. I have had the opportunity to give presentations to hundreds of school counselors on this topic, and I assure them that with training, they can make an accurate and thorough assessment of suicide risk and take appropriate action. Johnson and Maile (1987) comment that school personnel learn quickly and overcome their anxiety. I hope that this chapter will give them confidence and the direction to proceed, because I know that each secondary school counselor will be confronted with a suicidal student sooner or later.

I also know what counselors want, because they have told me: They want someone else to come make an assessment of the suicidal student, or a suicide assessment scale that tells them exactly what to do. A counselor at an in-service session asked me, "Isn't there a scale that adds up and then, depending on the number, you take certain actions?" The answer is that our assessment scales are not that precise. The teacher's manual published by the association known as the Samaritans (Fencik, 1986) states plainly, "There is not a reliable psychological test that will identify someone who is suicidal. The best way to find out is to ask. If the person trusts that he or she will not be ridiculed or be the target of anger, he or she will most likely give a truthful answer" (p. 23). Hoff (1978), in discussing the effectiveness of lethality assessment scales, has stated, "Most of these scales are not very effective" (p. 117). Hoff stresses the importance of communication in the assessment process and lists several goals of assessment: (1) to cut down the guesswork and reduce confusion, (2) to increase the appropriate utilization of hospital services, and (3) to lower the anxiety of the personnel working with the suicidal person. Davis et al. (1988), on the other hand, have more faith in psychological tests that assess suicide potential. They name the following three instruments as the most promising: the Hilson Adolescent Profile (Inwald, Brobst, & Morrisey, 1987), the Suicidal Ideation Questionnaire (Reynolds, 1987), and the Suicide Probability Scale (Cull & Gill, 1982). They do, however, caution that the validity of all three instruments hasn't been adequately tested to date.

There are very careful and concrete ways in which counselors can assess lethality. The assessment process involves asking a series of questions, which counselors can easily learn to do. A counselor once called me and said that a student was suicidal. I asked how the counselor knew this, and the counselor replied that a classmate had relayed the information. I asked whether the counselor had seen the student. The answer was no; seeing the student was what the counselor wanted me to do. I know that in a large high school it is a necessity that the school counselor be able to make initial inquiries about suicidal behavior. I reminded the counselor of the in-service session that he had attended, provided him with specific questions to ask the student, and gave him encouragement that he could do it. I also pointed out that the student knew the counselor and would be comfortable talking to him. I promised to stay by the phone to provide consultation after the student was seen. The counselor called back, and we discussed the situation at length. It was not necessary for me to see the student, and the counselor handled the situation well. This example illustrates some of counselors' uncertainty in this area.

Not enough attention has been focused on the role of the school in assessing the lethality of students' suicidal ideation. Capuzzi (1987) stresses that counselors must be ready and trained to handle suicidal students before a prevention program is started. The California State Board of Education (1987) makes no distinction between the caring inquiry of any faculty member and the assessment that a trained counselor can perform. The Wisconsin Department of Instruction (1986) addresses assessment only briefly, and also does not distinguish the counselor's role from that of other staff. It states that all staff members should pay attention to "SAL" (Specifics of the plan, Availability of a method, and Lethality of the method). Lennox (1987) asserts that the school is responsible for having someone trained to make a thorough assessment of lethality, and that the degree of lethality determines the need for outside referral. Lennox also notes the need for consultation services to be available for the counselor. This is a role with which I am very familiar, and one that the psychologists on my staff perform daily.

Ross (1985a) observes that counselors may have such difficulty confronting students about their suicidal actions that they can become immobilized and take one step forward and two backward. Barrett (1985b) lists three important personal issues that counselors must work on if they are to assist suicidal students effectively: Counselors' attitude towards death and suicide in particular must not interfere with their ability to be reasonably comfortable with the topic; they must be careful not to display anxiety or irritation to students; and they must deal with feelings of insecurity and seek out additional training and/or support in this area. Counselors may also fear making a decision about what to do to assist suicidal students. Barrett points out that counselors fear underreacting and not doing enough to sound the alarm that a student is suicidal; however, counselors can also overreact and unnecessarily alarm a student and his or her family. Barrett notes how important trust is to adolescents, and states that whether or not to alert parents is a judgment call based on the question of whether or not the student is in "clear danger." My recommendation is to notify the family. The question should be *what* we say to them, and not *whether* to call the family.

Barrett (1985b) recommends that every counselor receive training in this area so that he or she can get a clear clinical picture of the student and the crisis situation. Training should include child and adolescent development, identification and assessment of suicide potential, intervention strategies, ethical and liability issues, and identification of community resources. Barrett stresses the need for counselors to know their limitations, so that they can realize when to refer and when to seek collaboration on difficult cases. A careful and thorough approach is recommended, including record keeping. Barrett (1985b) has developed the Suicide Assessment and Intervention Form (SAIF). Barrett made a very key point that there is a distinction between "assessment" and "prediction." The purpose of assessment in the schools is to identify a course of action; we need not make predictions about the likelihood of suicide. The SAIF is used as an instrument to interview students, and its questions address several main areas:

1. What stress is the student under?
2. What is the student's current emotional state? What are the behavioral symptoms?
3. Is there a specific plan to commit suicide?
4. Has a place and time been identified?
5. Is rescue likely?
6. How lethal is the method?
7. Has the student publicly talked about suicide?
8. Is there a history of suicidal thoughts or attempts?
9. What resources or assistance does the student seek?
10. What action should be taken to assist the student?

Barrett (1985b) suggests that the counselor present himself or herself as a helper who encourages the student to express his or her feelings, and that the counselor and student together explore strategies to improve the crisis situation. Barrett comments that the student's confidence can be obtained by stating, "I have helped other young people who felt they wanted to end their lives and I feel that I can help you" (1985b, p. 70). Suicidal students need to trust the counselor and feel that the counselor truly cares.

Hipple (1983) emphasizes the need to inquire directly about suicidal behavior and plans. Particular attention should be paid to the specifics of the plan, the time frame, and the possibility of rescue. Hipple further recommends that the counselor take a thorough case history of the student. The counselor serves as clarifier, teacher, and encourager. Hipple notes the importance of the counselor's helping the student understand his or her motives for suicide, affirming the worth of the student, and pointing out that the student does not have to act on suicidal impulses. Eyeman (1987) recommends getting the student to focus on coping skills and other factors that have kept him or her alive, and emphasizing that the student has control over his or her suicidal thoughts. Eyeman suggests that counselors examine the frequency, intensity, and duration of the student's suicidal thoughts; whether there has been a precipitating event; and what the student hopes to gain by committing suicide. Barrett (1985b) points out that the anxiety that counselors experience may cause them to rush their assessment, and comments that this is counterproductive: "The assessment process should not be conducted hastily and the interviewer should be cognizant of his need to get it over with" (p. 69).

The pressure to manage a suicidal student can also cause the counselor to overlook underlying psychological dynamics (Eyeman, 1987).

The need for direct inquiry is noted by Bonner (1987):

> Our greatest key to understanding, intervening and preventing suicide is to *directly* inquire into suicidal thinking and behavior. The suicidal person knows best why it is being considered. Attempts to mark, hide, or avoid such inquiry in research, therapy and human exchange are ignorant and destructive. (p. 12)

Bonner stresses that thoughts of suicide are not planted in a student's head by conversation and inquiry. The relief that adolescents feel when someone recognizes their feelings and is willing to talk openly about them is stressed by Brown (1987). Brown also suggests some "do's" and "don'ts" for shelter personnel that have much relevance for the counselor. The "do's" are as follows:

1. Talk openly about suicide.
2. Show that you care and the adolescent is not alone.
3. Remain calm; proceed slowly.
4. Be positive.
5. Know your limits.
6. Clarify the permanence of death.
7. Emphasize alternatives.
8. Act quickly to help the adolescent.

Brown's "don'ts" are the following:

1. Being shocked.
2. Encouraging guilt.
3. Trying to physically take away a weapon.
4. Promising total confidentiality.
5. Arguing against suicide.
6. Minimizing the problem.
7. Leaving the client alone.
8. Getting overinvolved.
9. Giving up hope.

Garfinkel (1986) makes a number of recommendations for assessment when a suicide attempt has already occurred. The events of the 48 hours prior to the attempt should be reviewed with the student and examined to determine whether psychosocial stressors or a psychiatric disorder was the reason for the attempt. Garfinkel also recommends that the actual attempt should be examined; the assessment should include the following questions, which were formulated by Beck, Schuyler, and Herman (1974):

1. Were others near by, and what was the likelihood of rescue?
2. Were precautions taken to avoid discovery, and was a note left?
3. Were others told of the attempt before it happened?
4. Were others told of the attempt afterwards?
5. Is there a family history of suicide?

Garfinkel (1986) notes the need to establish a therapeutic alliance with the suicidal student, to identify the stressors the student is experiencing, and to determine what coping mechanisms and support systems are available. The counselor needs to take an advocate role and be available through every school day. Garfinkel is critical of several existing school suicide prevention programs; he feels that a psychiatrist needs to be a part of the school's suicide response team and that the comprehensive evaluation of a suicidal student should be based on a systematic psychiatric protocol.

Boggs (1987) cautions against trying to cheer up suicide attempters and recommends that schools not minimize the seriousness of the situation. Faculty members need to know when a student has attempted suicide, so that they will be able to dispel rumors and respond appropriately and supportively to the student. Smith (1985) gives examples of direct inquiry following an attempt and suggests the following questions:

- Did you intend to die?
- Who would have been affected?
- Did you dream of suicide?
- Would your family have been better off?

A calm, thorough interview with the suicidal student is recommended by McBrien (1983). The counselor should interview the student as if the student were planning a trip. McBrien describes the counselor's role thus: "When a student admits to having thoughts about suicide, the work of the counselor is to evaluate the seriousness of the threat and to decide whether to refer the student to local mental health resources, to begin continually counseling or to classify the student as nonsuicidal" (p. 79). The cognitions of the student are emphasized, and the strategy recommended is to confront the student directly, honestly, and openly. McBrien suggests asking 10 critical questions. I have found these questions to be helpful, and feel that the format of viewing the suicidal thoughts as if the student were taking a trip encourages the calmness and thoroughness McBrien recommends. McBrien states the purpose of the 10 questions as follows:

These ten questions serve as the data base for the decision to start the referral process for the high-risk student or to continue counseling the low-risk student. There is no cutoff score to rely on; it requires clinical judgement based on the training and experience of the counselor, especially empathy and active listening skills. (1983, p. 80)

McBrien also recommends that if a counselor feels confident he or she can work with a low-risk student, the student need not be referred elsewhere. I recommend that the student's parents still be informed. The questions that McBrien recommends are the following:

1. What are the specifics of the plan?
2. How much does the student want to die?
3. How much does the student want to live?
4. How often does the student have suicidal thoughts?
5. How long has the student had suicidal thoughts?
6. Is there a lifeline to stop the student?
7. Has the student made previous suicide attempts?
8. Has the student made final arrangements or chosen a time to die?
9. What is the chance that the student will kill himself or herself?
10. Why does the student want to die?

The last question is the one that we all want answered; McBrien recommends not asking it if a counselor is going to refer a student. I also caution against the counselor's getting into the "why," but instead recommend more attention to degree of lethality. School personnel are not going to be able to solve the problems that cause a young person to be suicidal, but they can set in motion a combined effort involving the student, his or her family, and community resources that can do so.

Lennox (1987) recommends that the counselor not make any deals with the student to keep secrets about suicidal behavior. Cantor (1985) makes a similar recommendation and adds, "I also tell my patients that if I feel they are in danger of taking their lives, I will not keep quiet" (p. 15).

Eyeman (1987) emphasizes the following key points not addressed by McBrien:

1. Does the suicidal person have control over his or her suicidal thoughts, and can he or she get rid of them?
2. What does he or she hope to gain from suicide?
3. Has there been a precipitating event?
4. Has the person thought about how others would react to his or her death?

5. Is there a past history of suicide in the family?
6. Is there a preoccupation with death?

Two questions that I also feel need to be added are these:

7. Is the student involved with drugs?
8. Does the student understand the finality of death?

Johnson and Maile (1987), like Boggs (1987), advise against the counselor's trying to rescue or cheer up the student or arguing against suicide. They recommend not trying to find out "why." The question of what to do if an adolescent refuses to answer questions about suicidal thoughts is addressed by Eyeman (1987), who recommends having the adolescent write out his or her thoughts.

A number of school districts attempt to classify suicidal adolescents into low-, medium-, or high-risk categories. One such classification system (J. Smith, 1988a) is used by the Dallas Independent School District and appears as Appendix D of this book. The specifics of the suicidal plan and the student's history, coping behavior, life style, and medical status are all considered across the continuum of low, medium, or high risk. I find this approach helpful, but caution counselors not to try to make an assessment turn out to indicate low risk so that parent contact can be avoided. There also is no cutoff score with such a method. Low-risk students have vague thoughts of hopelessness, but do not have plans to commit suicide using lethal methods. Medium-risk students have made direct statements about suicide, but do not have a detailed plan involving a lethal method close at hand. High-risk students have a detailed plan involving a lethal method: They have made final arrangements, decided that suicide is the only alternative, and thought about exactly when and how they will commit suicide.

The intervention for a low-risk student involves parent contact, but the discussion may not focus on suicide exclusively; instead, it should focus on the general mood of the student and on helping the student to increase his or her coping skills. The counselor should have the student sign a no-suicide contract (see the following section), give the student the local crisis hotline number, be available to the student for further consultation, and monitor the student closely.

The medium-risk student's parents must be contacted as soon as possible, and the focus of the contact should be on suicide. This student should also sign a no-suicide contract, and referral should be made to services in the community (in addition to the support and monitoring at school).

The high-risk student should be handled in the same way as the medium-risk student, except that he or she should not be left alone. An administrator should be notified, and parents should be told to come to school to pick up their child. All lethal instruments should be kept away from the student. Necessary community services may include hospitalization.

NO-SUICIDE CONTRACTS

McBrien (1983) strongly recommends that counselors use a no-suicide contract: "Suicidal thinking can be impulsive, and it is important that the student has control over such impulses. The no-suicide contract offers the control that the student needs" (p. 81). Barrett (1985b) stresses that such a contract can help reduce the student's anxiety. I have also found that it relieves the anxiety of the counselor. Hipple (1983) believes that the contract helps the student take control over his or her suicidal thoughts. McBrien notes that students feel relief after they have signed a contract and that the contract represents a commitment on their part to controlling their suicidal impulses and to counseling itself.

The question has been raised as to how effective contracts are in preventing youth suicide. McBrien (1983) reports a study in which 600 patients signed no-suicide contracts and not one committed suicide. I have had numerous students sign contracts with the same result. I have also monitored the results in our large school district for 7 years, and not one of the hundreds of students who signed a contract committed suicide. Some have attempted suicide, but none have completed it. One point that must be made is that a contract is not enough by itself. It is desirable and necessary, but does not take the place of parent contact. Barrett (1985b) comments, "The contract is a tool which should be used in conjunction with protective measures and never in isolation" (p. 76).

Counselors have asked what a no-suicide contract should contain. I recommend that each contract be tailor-made for the student and the circumstances, and written in the presence of the student. The most official-looking school stationery should be used. The contract should be signed by the student and the counselor, and the student should be given a copy. Some counselors prefer to have contracts typed up and ready to use. A sample contract appears below:

No-Suicide Contract

I, _____(name)_____ , a student at _____(school)_____ , take the responsibility for my welfare, and I agree not to harm myself in any way. I understand that if I am having suicidal thoughts, I agree to call my counselor, _____(name)_____ , at _(phone number)_ . If I cannot reach my counselor, I will call the crisis hotline at _(phone number)_ , or I will tell the nearest adult and get help for myself.

Specific details can be worked into this basic form to address the use of lethal instruments, whether the student is at school or home, or other unique circumstances, especially those related to impulsivity and substance use. It is also important to prepare students in the event that the crisis hotline number is busy. I make them promise to keep calling or tell the nearest adult.

Contracts can be used with students at almost any age. I have contracts with students as young as age 7. A child of 7 does not understand the concept of responsibility for one's own welfare as clearly as an older student does; however, the no-suicide contract is a concrete activity that the counselor and student can do together to further their alliance. The contract also is not the only thing that I recommend.

Sometimes students refuse to sign a no-suicide contract. This can cause much anxiety for the counselor. What should be done? The following case example deals with such a situation.

J, a 15-year-old boy, was referred to me after he left a suicide note in class. An extensive interview indicated no pattern of suicide in the family. J had made no previous attempt, but had made previous threats of suicide. He also had a history of school and family problems, and had recently broken up with his girlfriend. He had a specific plan to jump off the nearby Hyatt Hotel and stated that he had been on the roof the day before. J was at high risk for suicide; however, he refused to sign the no-suicide contract, commenting, "If I sign this, then I can't follow through on my plan to commit suicide." I stated that this was correct and again asked him to sign. He again refused. I kept the student with me while I called his mother; at my request, she came to the school immediately. J and his mother went to see a private practitioner that afternoon, and J was hospitalized. His refusal to sign the contract heightened his suicide risk and made it essential that I supervise him closely until his parents assumed responsibility for him.

We must inquire directly about suicidal thoughts. I do not hesitate to ask, "Have you thought about how you would end your life or how you would kill yourself?" Sometimes students reply, "No, I haven't thought about how; I just know my life is hopeless." One student answered that he would jump off a cliff. I wasn't too alarmed, as the Houston area is one of the flattest places on earth, but I had him sign a contract and I called his parents. Another student once responded, "I'd use a .38 pistol. I have it at home, and I had it out last night." I not only had this student sign a contract, but kept him with me until his parents came to the school.

There is no exact statement or phrase that should be used in questioning a suicidal student. It is important for us to remember that we are making an assessment of lethality to guide our actions to assist students. We are not trying to solve their problems in one session, nor are we trying to make a prediction about their likelihood of suicide. Instead, we are trying to gather information that will help us know what to say to parents, how much supervision to provide the students, and whether or not services from the community are needed. Table 5.3 outlines the basic approach that a counselor should employ.

I strongly recommend that counselors rehearse asking students questions about suicide. I have had counselors ask me to demonstrate this on numerous occasions. Heiman et al. (1985) feel that it is important for school personnel to role-play the questioning of students, and they also emphasize the importance of calling a colleague to get a second opinion on a particular case. Heiman et al. comment, "As school staff began to view assessment and intervention as a skill that can be acquired, they become more confident in their own ability to be effective" (p. 267). Counselors can role-play with each other, or they can ask drama students to role-play with them. Counselors must understand that by inquiring directly about suicide, they will not cause a student to commit suicide. A student who is not suicidal will simply let the counselor know that suicide is not a problem for him or her. A counselor with whom I work once commented, "I have learned to ask students about suicidal thoughts. It isn't as scary as it used to be." It is essential today that school personnel, especially school counselors, have confidence in their ability to work openly and directly on this topic.

SUICIDE ATTEMPTS AT SCHOOL

The California State Department of Education (1987) recommends treating a suicide attempt at school as a psychiatric and medical emergency. First aid and medical assistance may be needed. If poisoning is suspected, then school personnel should identify what the substance was and how much was ingested. The principal needs to be notified immediately, and police or paramedics should be called to transport the student to the hospital. The principles recommended in the chapter on postvention (see Chapter 8) should be followed to dispel rumors.

TABLE 5.3. Guidelines to Counselors for Assessing Lethality and Assisting a Suicidal Student

- Be aware of your personal issues on this topic.
- Calmly gather information to assess lethality and to identify a course of action.
- Listening skills are very important. Reflect feelings, be nonjudgmental, and avoid minimizing the problem.
- Ideally, you should already have a relationship with the student.
- Communicate caring, support, and trust, while providing encouragement that the student can cope.
- Inquire directly about suicidal plans, method, time, and place.
- Emphasize the student's worth and his or her previous coping skills. Be hopeful.
- Gather information about the student's history, with emphasis on the suicidal history of the student and family and on substance use.
- Has anyone been told about suicidal plans, and what is the possibility of rescue?
- Has the student made any final arrangements?
- Has the student imagined the reaction of others to his or her death?
- Does the student understand the finality of death?
- Keep notes of your interaction with the student.
- Do not leave medium- or high-risk students alone.
- Have the student sign a no-suicide contract. If the student refuses to sign, stay with him or her.
- Get supportive collaboration from a colleague.
- Let the student know the limits of confidentiality, and explain why it is in the student's best interest to inform parents so everyone can work together to assist him or her.
- Be familiar with community resources.
- Outline for the student the steps that are being taken to help him or her.
- Emphasize alternatives to suicide.
- Make a follow-up appointment with the student.
- Notify the parents of the student.

CARE FOR THE CAREGIVER

The term "care for the caregiver" has been used by several writers (e.g., Barrett, 1985b; Brown, 1987). Much has been written about the stress and anxiety that counselors feel when dealing with suicidal students. Brown and Schroff (1986) have made several suggestions to help counselors take care of themselves:

1. Get the opinion and support of others.
2. Recognize that you cannot assume the responsibility for the life of the student.

3. This process may cause you to have intense feelings that you need to process with colleagues.
4. Clarify your feelings about suicide.

Barrett (1985b) also stresses the intense emotions that may be aroused, as well as the inadequacy feelings. One of the most productive things that secondary school counselors can do is to recognize the likelihood that they will be working with suicidal students and to prepare themselves through attending workshops, reading books and journal articles, exploring their personal experiences on the topic, and rehearsing lethality assessment. Processing the specifics of the situation and getting a second opinion are also recommended. Assessing lethality should be a joint effort by two or more professionals. Many school counselors with whom I work have their secretaries supervise suicidal students while they excuse themselves for a few minutes and call me for a consultation. Most of the time, the counselors have thought of all the right questions and just need someone to encourage them and tell them they can handle it.

As caretakers in the schools, we must recognize that there are limits to what we can do and that much of the outcome for suicidal students is the responsibility of the students and their families. We must process, debrief, do things to be good to ourselves, and look for a glimmer of humor in the situation. A team of counselors was once working with a suicidal student, unbeknownst to one counselor. The counselor who did not know what was going on had his mind on eating the cheesecake that had been brought in that morning. He interrupted the conference about suicide and asked, "Shall I get the knife?" He meant for the cheesecake, but didn't say so. This was not received with humor at the time, but after the student was assisted and the parent was contacted it became a source of amusement.

A group of high school counselors can alleviate much of their stress by eating lunch together each day. Cases are discussed, frustrations are shared, and support is received.

CONFIDENTIALITY

One of the basic premises of this book, and of suicide prevention in general, is that we must not keep secrets about suicidal behavior. This premise applies to all who come in contact with a suicidal student, whether they are friends, classmates, teachers, or counselors. Liability can be an issue for the school district and for individual counselors. Counselors can leave themselves open to liability damages if they keep secrets about suicidal behavior.

I acknowledge that students expect confidentiality in a counseling relationship; however, the key point is that whenever the welfare of a minor is at stake, as is the case with a suicidal student, then the parents must be notified. The ideal situation for school counselors is to have gone over the limits of confidentiality with students in advance. I use a form that explains that limits do exist concerning the information that is shared in counseling. I recommend that counselors use such a form. However, if such a form is not signed, the same confidence limits still exist. A counselor obviously does not want to curtail a student's discussion of suicidal thoughts by immediately bringing up the issue of confidentiality. My recommendation is to get the most complete information possible about the student's suicidal thoughts and plans first, and then to deal directly with the limit of confidentiality. The reality is that information about suicidal behavior can and must be revealed when the student is under 18 years of age.

The issue of confidentiality has been addressed by the Indiana State Board of Health (1985). The board's guide to suicide prevention states, in part, "Youngsters often will share highly sensitive, personal matters with adults if they 'promise not to tell anyone.' It is easy and very tempting to enter into such an agreement; however, taking this approach is very dangerous" (p. 27).

The counselor must break confidentiality concerning suicidal behavior. The next question the counselor must address is that of who needs to know about the suicidal behavior. I recommend that, at a minimum, the school administration and the parents need to know. A school psychologist in Chicago was recently suspended for failing to disclose information concerning the suicidal statements of a student (Spittzzeri, 1987). The school district felt that the school psychologist had a duty to advise the school administration. The school psychologist took the matter to the court, which ruled in favor of the school district. Doyle (1987) stresses that for all intents and purposes, there is no privileged communication between students and licensed professionals practicing in the schools:

> The reason is that the relationship is viewed as being between the school and the student, not between the student and the licensed professional. There is also a duty of the licensed professional to report to the school administrator and the information in the school records is not privileged. (p. 3)

Doyle recommends that the parents or guardian be notified if a student under the age of 18 years of age is suicidal. Doyle stresses that the principal needs to know even when the student is 18, as do the other educators who have a legitimate interest in the student. School staff members who have responsibility for the student need to know when a student is suicidal (Ruof et al., 1987).

I agree with Doyle's recommendations. I especially think that it is important that we keep school administrators informed about suicidal behavior. Much has been written concerning the reluctance of school administrators to recognize the problem of youth suicide and work on it. How can we expect them to work on the problem when we withhold information from them about its occurrence? School administrators must be part of the school response team and must play a supportive role to the counselor or school psychologist, not an adversarial one as in the case in Chicago. The question of what to do about notifying a student's parents when the student is 18 years of age is a gray area. I recommend that they be notified. I believe that students who are approached directly and honestly about the limits of confidentiality will understand that what is being done is in their best interest.

PARENT NOTIFICATION

The question is not whether to call the parents of a suicidal student, but instead how to elicit a supportive reaction from the parents. Parents must be notified. The notification may need to be immediate and in person, depending on the student's level of risk. Parents may react with disbelief, or they may focus on their own needs by saying something like "How could my child do this to me?" Parents should logically be notified by the counselor who assesses lethality. The counselor needs to be calm, assertive, and thorough. It may be necessary to repeat phrases several times, to give the parents an explanation of how the counselor arrived at the conclusion that their child is suicidal, and to describe the credentials or experience qualifying the counselor to make such a determination. The phone call to parents or the conference to disclose this type of information is very stressful for counselors, and I recommend that a counselor have the assistance of a colleague or administrator. Johnson and Maile (1987) have suggested the following guidelines for the parents of suicidal youths:

1. Be patient with the child.
2. Take threats and gestures seriously.
3. Show them love, acceptance, and tolerance, and seek out the help they need.
4. Keep communication going and avoid isolation.
5. Offer help with no strings attached.

Together, these points constitute an excellent goal for the type of reaction that the counselor wants to elicit from the parents. Parents need to understand the seriousness of the problem and the importance of acting quickly. School counselors have commented that suicidal crises often develop late in the school day, which creates quite a dilemma about supervision. Lennox (1987) cautions against sending a suicidal student home to an empty house and recommends that if the parents refuse to get help for the child, then child welfare services need to be called.

A number of recommendations for parent notification have been made by Barrett (1985b), who emphasizes examining the relationship between the parents and the child. The counselor should look at how the child is viewed in the family, determine whether or not the parents seem depressed, and evaluate their willingness to follow the counselor's recommendations. Parents often state that the student is only trying to get attention or manipulate adults. I acknowledge that this may be the case; however, I agree with Barrett (1985b), who stresses that this is not a time for parents to get tough. Professional assistance is needed whenever a child attempts to manipulate others through suicidal behavior.

One parent whom I called recently was not surprised by the call and said, "I have been expecting the school to call, as I have been waiting for the other shoe to drop." The parent went on to tell me about two previous attempts the girl had made. The parent had not taken the girl for treatment, but did agree to do so after our conference. I wondered what might have happened if the school had not detected the suicidal behavior.

It is important to avoid keeping secrets from students about the conversation with their parents. I give suicidal students the opportunity to make the call with myself in the room. If they decline, then I make the call and let them listen. Some students try to get me to let them go home, so they can tell their parents on their own; my response is a firm no. A major concern for students is that their parents will go crazy and yell at them or even punish them. I respond by saying that I have had experience at this and will do my best to elicit a supportive reaction from their parents. One mother who came to school responded by telling her daughter, "Don't you ever talk this way again!" The mother wanted to wipe out her daughter's suicidal thoughts. I encouraged the mother to talk less and listen more, and pointed out that it was positive that her daughter was expressing these thoughts. I urge parents to "reach out" to their children and avoid preaching to them. There are three rules of communication for the parents of a suicidal child—listen, listen, listen! Suicidal thoughts will not go away because parents wish them to or because parents order their children not to think about suicide.

The goal of parent contact is to help a student by setting in motion steps to work on the student's long-standing problems. Ideally, a transfer of the role of primary caretaker from the school counselor to a caretaker in the community should take place. In addition, parents need to be accepting and nurturing, to increase their supervision, and to remove any readily available lethal instruments. Ruof et al. (1987) stress the necessity of informing parents. They recommend that the student be informed that notification will take place and that two school staff members conduct the notification conference. If parents do not respond or fail to see the severity of the situation, then child welfare services should be contacted, as it is neglectful not to provide treatment for a suicidal child. I have found that mentioning the possibility of calling the child welfare agency convinces almost all parents to follow through on treatment recommendations. A number of school districts have parents sign a form verifying that they have been notified of the suicidal risk of their child. Such forms can be used very effectively to document that the parents were notified. An example of an emergency verification form appears as Appendix E of this book.

Ruof and Harris (1988a) address the question of how far the school should go to secure services for the student. Schools are not liable for hospital bills when students are taken to the hospital. On the issue of confidentiality and responsibility, Ruof and Harris comment,

> The bottom line [is] that if the child's right to be in a safe situation conflicts with the parent's right to confidentiality, the child's right to be safeguarded takes precedence. Our policy states that schools are in the position and have the duty to make appropriate referrals on suicidal students and secure assistance for them. (1988a, p. 18)

Stanton and Stanton (1987) make the following suggestions for helping the parents of suicidal adolescents:

1. Parents need to be empowered to help the adolescent.
2. Parental strengths need to be found and reinforced.
3. Parents need to work together.
4. A home safety watch should be implemented.

Stanton and Stanton point out that the home safety watch helps parents feel competent and useful and may avoid hospital expenses. They comment, "Therapy that weakens parents can increase the risk of death. Therapy that supports and empowers parents then can help save lives" (1987, p. 3).

Parental notification is a very complicated process, and several case examples are offered here to illustrate its complexities. S, a 16-year-old student, stated that he had thought of suicide and had access to a shotgun. He commented, "I loaded it, put the gun in my mouth, and put my big toe on the trigger." I insisted that his mother come for a conference. She did so, but said such things as, "He doesn't know where the gun or the ammunition is." I insisted that he did, and recommended that an appointment be made with the family therapist whom the student had previously seen. The mother called the therapist and made an appointment; she also agreed to take the gun out of the house. I gave the mother a copy of the no-suicide contract that the student had signed. I encouraged the mother to be supportive and to focus on her son's needs. The mother and I then informed the student, who was being supervised by my secretary, of what steps were being taken. I scheduled a follow-up appointment with the student.

R, a 15-year-old student, was awaiting trial for manslaughter. He stated that he planned to hang himself that evening and had prepared the noose the night before. He did not want his parents called, but, after a discussion, he agreed that it was in his best interest. His father at first refused to come to the school and commented, "It might be for the best if my son went ahead and killed himself after all the trouble he caused." I calmly assured him that I knew how upsetting this information was, and I knew that he didn't mean what he said. He eventually agreed to come to school to pick up his son, but refused to seek outside counseling for the son. I notified the child welfare department.

Most of the parents I have notified have reacted positively and have followed through on recommendations. Their initial reaction is often shock or denial. I sometimes talk with the parents privately and then bring in the student. It is very important that no secrets be kept, and it is recommended that both parents be involved if at all possible. I have had parents become quite angry and claim that I am exaggerating the situation. One father even had his son call me after our conference to tell me that the son had made up everything that he told me about suicidal behavior. The father did not follow through on my recommendations, so I called the child welfare agency. I also sent the father a letter stating the seriousness of the situation and reiterated my recommendations. The issue of what to do when parents minimize the seriousness of their child's plight and do not seek help for the child is a frustrating one. The AAS is working on this issue.

What happens when parents refuse to get involved or are unreachable, and the counselor must deal with a suicidal student without an active parent or guardian? R, a 17-year-old student who was not living with his parents, attempted suicide by running in front of a car. His parents could not be reached. One of the psychologists for the school district testified before a judge and had a mental health warrant served on R, which resulted in his being transferred to the county psychiatric hospital.

What happens when parents refuse to take firearms or other weapons out of the house after being notified that their child has made plans to use those weapons to commit suicide? On one occasion, a psychologist who could not reach parents went to the home with the sister of the suicidal student and removed the guns. On another occasion, an assistant principal and a psychologist went to the home and talked a suicidal student into putting down knives and coming with them to school. Parents must understand the importance of removing lethal weapons from the home when their child is suicidal. The *Houston Post* (March 5, 1988) reported a note left by a teenage girl who shot herself, which warned her parents not to leave a gun in the house.

Another student who convinced us of his immediate plans to commit suicide was transported in an assistant principal's van to a nearby psychiatric hospital. I remember this situation very well, because I sat between the student and the door and was prepared to grab him if he tried to jump out. His mother met us at the hospital, and he was admitted. We have also arranged for suicidal students to be picked up by a family friend or neighbor when we could not reach parents. Staff members have also stayed late at school with suicidal students until parents could come to school. One father wanted us to let his son drive his car home and said that he would meet his son at home. We insisted that the father come to school and follow his son home.

Parents have also requested that school psychologists and counselors not talk with their children again. Our district policy is that when a student is in crisis or has been a discipline problem, we dispense with obtaining parental permission before the psychologist sees a student. Parents are informed afterwards. Texas has recently passed Senate Bill 1122, which authorizes professionals to provide services to a minor without parental consent under certain conditions, one of which is suicide prevention. A parent who requested that her daughter not be seen again by the school psychologist was told that we could and would see her any time that we believed her to be suicidal, in accordance with Senate Bill 1122.

What happens when parents are willing to seek treatment for their child but have no money or insurance to do so? The school district where I am employed pays for a one-time consultation with community mental health professionals. Parents are made aware that the district cannot pay for ongoing treatment. This option has proved very valuable both in transferring responsibility to the community and in locating more assistance for students. In addition, we utilize the limited state and county resources that are available.

Recommendations for parent notification appear in Table 5.4.

REFERRAL TO COMMUNITY SERVICES

The community services to which suicidal students are referred should be professionals or agencies that have experience in treating suicidal youths. They also need to have proven to work cooperatively with the school district and to provide feedback and suggestions to the district. Colt (1986) notes that psychiatrists are viewed as being the authorities on treating suicidal patients; however, he points out that all psychiatrists may not have been trained adequately, nor do they have the desire to work with suicidal patients. School personnel need to know the skills and interests of the private practitioners or agencies to which referrals are made. These sources need to be readily available to assist, due to the

---

TABLE 5.4. Goals and Procedures for Notifying Parents of Suicidal Behavior

- Parents must be notified; a conference at school is preferable to telephone notification.
- Two school staff members should be involved, as should both parents (if at all possible), and a cooperative effort to help the student should be emphasized.
- Parents should be made to understand the severity of the situation and should be provided with suggestions to increase supervision, reduce the availability of lethal weapons, and assist their child.
- The student should be included in all or part of the conference.
- Parents may be requested to sign a form acknowledging that they have been notified that their child is suicidal (see Appendix E).
- A referral to a mental health professional in the community who has access to hospitalization is almost certainly needed.
- A release-of-information form should be signed, so that communication between the community mental health professional and the school can take place.
- Follow-up services at school should be discussed and an appointment made with the student.
- Parents should be requested to keep the school informed about the outside treatment.
- Parents who refuse to follow the school's recommendations should be told that the child welfare agency will be called, and the school personnel should not hesitate to do so. A follow-up letter should be mailed to parents.
- Assistance at school should be provided to the student, no matter what the reaction of the parents is, in accordance with local and state guidelines.

---

importance of acting quickly to assist the student. Access to hospitalization and the fees charged by the professional or agency are all factors of which school personnel need to be aware. It is important that a cooperative relationship exist among the school personnel, the parents, and the community mental health professional, so that maximum support and assistance can be provided to a student. The school personnel who have made the referral must stay active with the student, and not completely turn over all support and treatment to the community mental health professional.

DISCIPLINE AND THE SUICIDAL STUDENT

Schools need to be very careful about suspending or expelling suicidal students. There have been students who have attempted and completed suicide following suspension. The key point is that school personnel notify parents and provide supervision to suicidal students who are being disciplined. In-school suspension is preferable to out-of-school suspension. Suicidal students simply should not be sent home for discipline. Their parents need to come to school, and personnel need to confer with them according to parent notification procedures. Ruof et al. (1987) provide an example of a form that combines suspension procedures with notification of suicidality. The form is given to the parents in person, along with specific recommendations about supervision and treatment. Suspension or expulsion can serve as a precipitating event, and appropriate precautions should be taken. Ruof and Harris (1988b) emphasize that limits must be set for school behavior, or suicidal students will feel even more out of control.

RURAL SCHOOLS

Small and rural school districts should have a suicide intervention program with written procedures, just as large urban districts should. The faculty members need to learn the warning signs and the referral procedures. Obviously, rural schools have fewer staff members to select to train in assessment; a rural school that does not have a counselor should train a nurse or an administrator to do the assessment. Resources in the nearest urban center should be identified and researched prior to a suicidal crisis. There may be a crisis hotline number that can be called toll-free. A consultant may be brought in to train school personnel and assist in developing and implementing an intervention program. I have provided such services to small school districts and have found them quite capable of implementing programs, although a small school district may be less likely to add a suicide awareness component to the curriculum. Small schools are not immune from a contagion effect, and the suicide of a student in a small community will receive extensive media attention, especially from the local newspaper.

SPECIAL EDUCATION MODEL

The role of special education has been addressed by Guetzloe (1988), who emphasizes that special education personnel have a responsibility to plan and implement suicide intervention programs. Guetzloe comments, "Exceptional children are often more vulnerable to emotional trauma which may lead to stress, feelings of low self-esteem and suicidal behavior" (1988, p. 25). Children with learning difficulties are at a higher risk for depression and suicidal behavior than normal children. Guetzloe recommends an active role for school special education personnel, even though not all suicidal children qualify for special education services. The knowledge and abilities of special education personnel are important resources for intervention. A few of these are observation skills, the ability to work with parents, intervention skills, working relationships with mental health professionals, and emphasis on a positive school environment.

Guetzloe also addresses the question of whether or not depressed children will qualify as seriously emotionally disturbed under federal guidelines. Depression is listed as a characteristic of seriously emotionally disturbed children. Guetzloe comments,

> However, the depression must be exhibited to a marked degree over a long period of time and must adversely affect educational performance in order to qualify a child for special education services. Because the definition is imprecise and the accompanying conditions are subject to interpretation, children who exhibit symptoms of depression may not be diagnosed as seriously emotionally disturbed. (1988, p. 26)

A collaborative effort between regular education and special education personnel is recommended. Guetzloe notes that the Minneapolis Public Schools utilize such an approach and provide a comprehensive special education assessment to students who are identified as suicidal. This is only one of the steps that should be taken to assist the suicidal child. This assessment process should be lengthy and should provide limited immediate assistance. I agree with these recommendations, and special education personnel can be very valuable in intervention efforts. Special education and regular education personnel need to cooperate and provide needed support and services to suicidal students, whether they are handicapped or not. Suicidal crises are one of the few situations in which school psychologists are allowed to work with regular education students. School psychologists have many skills to offer in suicide intervention and in creating more positive school climates, which would reduce the likelihood of suicide.

INVOLVEMENT OF PARENT ORGANIZATIONS AND COMMUNITY OUTREACH

Parent organizations can be a tremendous resource to a school district in both implementing and maintaining a suicide prevention program. The national PTA organization has been very involved at the national, state, and local levels in support of suicide prevention in the schools. Ann Kahn, the national PTA president, has commented, "It has been said that when you lose a parent you lose the past, but when you lose a child, you lose the future. It is a very serious commitment to try and reduce the number of children that we lose to youth suicide" (1985, p. 200). The PTA is committed to educating parents and school districts about suicide prevention. The state PTA in Texas supported the youth suicide prevention legislation.

The PTA has been very supportive of suicide prevention in the Fairfax County (Virginia) Public Schools. In 1987, the Fairfax County school system published a manual entitled *The Adolescent Suicide Prevention Program*, which contains information on parent involvement. Parents were invited to be represented on the district advisory board to develop the program. The advisory board works with all school PTA organizations, which sponsor and coordinate presentations to parents that are held throughout the year. The presentations are a joint effort of school staff and community mental health professionals. It has been my own experience that parental attendance at evening presentations on suicide prevention is small. The mother of B (see Chapter 3) commented after her son's suicide, "I knew that the school district made presentations on this topic, but I just didn't think that I needed to attend." The Fairfax County program encourages school district personnel to attend these sessions, to reinforce the idea that they are important. Parental resistance to the subject of suicide has been encountered as a result of fear and misinformation. The Fairfax County guide comments,

> Unfortunately, some parents remain resistant to the subject of suicide, finding it too distressing to comprehend. They did not readily agree to cooperate

in presenting the subject to other parents nor, in some cases, were they enthusiastic about having their children exposed to the topic. Efforts to reach this group have been continued. (Fairfax County Public Schools, 1987, p. 28)

Fairfax County has attempted to overcome this resistance by focusing on student stress and teaching problem-solving skills for students.

The school district should assume a leadership role to call youth suicide to the attention of the community. My district publishes a news-letter that is mailed to all parents and has featured suicide prevention on three occasions in recent years. The articles have stressed what parents should look for, how to respond to their children, and how the school district can help. Vidal (1986) comments, "If the family knows that a school has a helpful, nonthreatening manner of dealing with suicides, it is more likely to reveal that a son or daughter made an attempt" (p. 69). It is vitally important that school personnel know of such attempts and that cooperation exist between parents and school personnel. I recommend a series of parent presentations throughout the year at various secondary schools. Some of the most successful presentations that we have done have involved local members of the clergy.

We have also received favorable coverage from area newspapers, and headlines have emphasized that the district is "battling teen suicide." The information that parents need to prevent suicide is essentially the same information that school staff and students themselves need. An examina-tion of the California program (California State Department of Educa-tion, 1987) shows little difference in the information provided to the various groups. Everybody needs to know what to look for and how to respond. Every effort should be made to keep parents informed and involved in prevention efforts. I do not feel that nonsupportive parents should be allowed to stop a district from implementing a suicide preven-tion program. School staff members must be trained, with or without parental support. I also have reservations about the model proposed in Florida (described by Harris & Crawford, 1987), which would require parental permission before a student could be exposed to this informa-tion in the curriculum. Students need this information, and I think that school administrators should decide whether it is needed, not parents.

School district personnel can also provide much assistance to other professionals in the community. Ryerson (1988) recommends coordinat-ing the school program with the efforts of police officers, physicians, the clergy, and community mental health professionals. Cooperative train-ing meetings with these professionals are very important. I have had the opportunity to provide training on suicide prevention to the staff of the most popular radio station for teenagers in the Houston area. The staff members were very interested in knowing how to handle crisis calls and what they could do to help with this problem.

THE SCHOOL LIBRARY

A very basic question is this: What materials are available concerning youth suicide in the school library? There are a number of good books for teenagers on this topic. The Youth Suicide National Center has a list of recommended books for teens. The librarian needs to be familiar with youth suicide for several reasons. First, he or she needs to know what to look for when selecting books for the library on this topic. The books that deal directly with the topic should emphasize prevention; in particular, they should contain specific examples of how one teen can intervene and get help for a suicidal friend. Information about warning signs and sources of help is also important. All books should be reviewed before being placed in the library, and those that portray youth suicide in a mystic, romantic, or sensationalized way are not recommended.

The librarian should also find out why students want to read about this subject or do a report on it. Students who exhibit some of the warning signs should be referred, following school policy. A librarian who does not know a particular student who is checking out books on suicide should simply contact the grade-level counselor and let him or her know. The library should also contain a variety of books and articles on topics such as coping, problem solving, managing emotions, and maintaining a healthy life style.

I have reviewed books for librarians and made recommendations about whether they should or should not not be in the library. I have also been called by parents who were upset about the topic their child was researching. I am all for students' having information on this subject that is age-appropriate, factual, and preventive. We must also examine the history, stressors, and overall mental health of those students who are interested in this topic. I encourage librarians, as I do all members of the school staff, to trust their judgment and to be alarmists and seek help if they are concerned about a student.

STATUS OF SCHOOL PREVENTION PROGRAMS

There has been increasing interest in prevention efforts in the schools. How many school prevention programs are there, and what are their main components? Ryerson (1988) has described the development of school-based programs across the nation as a "grassroots" effort: There were only a handful of programs in 1980, and at the time of Ryerson's writing there were more than 114. Harris and Crawford (1987) found very few programs in place in the Texas schools. Columbia University researchers have been studying the effects of three school suicide prevention programs in New Jersey. The CDC in Atlanta, in collaboration with Columbia researchers, has been collecting data on the dates and places of teenagers' suicides for the past 8 years. It is noteworthy that research is being conducted, but as Berman (1987b) has pointed out, the amount of money allocated for such research is miniscule. Berman stresses that more emphasis should be placed on learning about adolescent coping skills.

The AAS has been gathering information about the status of school programs. A task force known as Wing Spread has had several meetings to study suicide programs in the schools. Berman (1986) has emphasized that Wing Spread is a national effort to develop a model school program and that serious attention will be given to behavior outcome measures to determine the effectiveness of school programs. The task force surveyed known school-related suicide programs in the schools in the United States and Canada. Questionnaires were mailed to 296 participants, and 158 were returned. The results of this survey are contained in the *Report of the School Suicide Programs Questionnaire* (Smith, Eyeman, Dyck, & Ryerson, 1987), which found the following:

1. Over half the programs were funded at least in part by public tax dollars.

2. Classroom approaches began on the average in the sixth grade, with the majority using an integrated curriculum that each program developed.

3. The most emphasis was placed on increasing student knowledge about suicide and getting help. Programs on the average took 3.5 hours.

4. Classroom time was allotted for lecture (39.6%), discussion (30.7%), films (15.4%), and experiential exercises (13.1%).

5. A number of programs (37.2%) did not have established referral procedures, and 37.3% did not have written evaluation procedures.

6. Training for school personnel, emphasizing detection of suicidal students, was reported by about one-third of the programs (32.5%).

7. Peer support programs that were non-classroom-based and emphasized students' befriending and helping others were reported by 24.6% of the participants.

8. The majority (72.8%) reported some form of crisis intervention program, with direct attention to students taking 42.5 of the total time. More of the crisis work was done by school personnel (58.9%) than by outside experts (41.1%).

9. Differences were found between American and Canadian programs. Canadian programs all had curriculum components, but fewer had peer support programs. Canadian programs were also more educational, whereas American programs combined educational and crisis intervention components.

The report raises a number of questions and cautions that more emphasis should be placed on evaluation. Its authors comment, "We must be mindful that however well intended, our efforts could be harmful and we need to know if and when that occurs and why" (Smith et al., 1987, p. 16). The report also raises the question of whether enough supervision is provided to peer support programs. Smith et al. conclude the report by noting that the increase in school programs is the result of the increase in the youth suicide rate and that the AAS has the responsibility to develop minimum standards for content supervision and program evaluation for schools.

The AAS appears to be moving slowly on these recommendations for schools, and a criticism has been that the initial Wing Spread task force did not, by intent, include anyone currently working in the schools. I am confident that very valuable recommendations will be made to the schools; however, there may be a problem in getting the information to those who work in the schools, as so few school personnel are AAS members. Major public relations efforts need to be aimed at all school personnel and their various organizations by the AAS.

EVALUATION OF SCHOOL PREVENTION PROGRAMS

A number of researchers have made recommendations concerning the evaluation of school prevention programs. The very existence of such programs has been questioned, for two reasons. The first seems to be the argument that having a prevention program somehow itself triggers or causes suicidal behavior. The second is the question of whether school prevention programs can be translated into the actual prevention of suicide.

The first of these issues has been dealt with at some length earlier in this chapter (see "Overview of the School's Role") and is discussed further below. On the second question, opinions differ. Shaffer (1988) emphasizes that prevention programs in the schools are the logical response, but cannot be assumed to be effective. Boggs (1987), however, cites a study that found high school students more able to detect suicidal behavior after a curriculum presentation. Ross (1985a) and Berman (1987b) have both cautioned that we cannot be certain that teaching a teenager the warning signs will actually translate into life-saving intervention with a friend; by contrast, Peck (1985) quotes a number of teenagers who felt they translated information into life-saving intervention.

Garland (1987) has summarized the preliminary results of the research being done at Columbia, which is funded by a National Institute of Mental Health grant. She notes that a recent newspaper headline reported that students were rejecting suicide prevention programs; Garland stresses that the headline exaggerated the Columbia group's findings. Suicide attempters did respond less favorably to curriculum suicide prevention programs than nonattempters, but their overall view of such programs was favorable. Preliminary results found that depression, antisocial tendencies, drug usage, and family history of suicide were linked to teenage suicide. The suicide of a family member was a factor approximately 33% of the time. Garland also notes that the diagnostic criteria of depression or conduct disorder could be applied approximately 80% of the time to suicidal students.

Berman (1987b) has cited the need for evaluation of school programs, noting that 40% had no evaluation component at all. A key component is to change the behavior of students so that they intervene to assist suicidal friends. Ryerson (1987) stresses the need for long-term studies to evaluate the effectiveness of school programs. The information about the warning signs of suicide must be translated into action by teenagers to assist suicidal friends. This point is also made in the *Report of the School Suicide Programs Questionnaire*, which states, "We should also encourage [that] evaluation criteria be more substantially related to our primary goals of changing behavior rather than assessing whether students can repeat what they are being taught" (Smith et al., 1987, p. 17). Ryerson (1987) has emphasized that most of the existing school programs are in suburbia, and that standard guidelines need to be developed as to what constitutes a good prevention program so that the information can be disseminated. Diane Ryerson and Judie Smith are the cochairs of the School Program Committee of the AAS, and I asked them informally why the organization does not officially recognize an outstanding school prevention program. Their response was that the AAS is not as yet ready to do so because there is considerable debate about what a school prevention program should consist of.

Ryerson (1987) has outlined the following basic components that she believes should be included in the evaluation of a school program:

1. The goals of the program should be defined.
2. Goals for outcome variables should be operationalized.

3. A homogeneous comparison or control group, which does not participate in the prevention program, should be located.
4. Outcome variables should be measured to determine the effectiveness of the program.

It seems likely that operational goals for a school prevention program would be to raise student and faculty awareness of suicidal behavior and to reduce suicides and suicide attempts. Garland (1987) cautions that severe attempts should be separated from suicidal gestures in evaluating the effectiveness of the program. One of the basic questions is that of where school personnel can get complete and accurate information about suicides and severe attempts. This information is not readily available. The Columbia researchers collected information from hospital emergency rooms. Another source of information would be the city or county coroner's office. The question of translating knowledge about the warning signs into intervention with a friend has mostly been evaluated by ratings on a survey. Schools need to document when students actually take steps to assist their suicidal friends. An example of this occurred while I was at my office on a Sunday morning working on this chapter. A high school girl called, asking for help for her suicidal friend. I complimented her on her response and provided assistance. I also added documentation of information being translated into action.

Barrett (1985a) has provided evaluative information about the Cherry Creek (Colorado) school-based suicide prevention program. Barrett reported that over 6,000 students participated in the curriculum-based suicide prevention project. The evaluation of the project found that students reported an increase in their basic knowledge of the warning signs and felt more confident to intervene to assist a suicidal friend. Barrett comments, "There has not been an increase in suicide or suicide attempts among this population of students. In fact, no suicides have occurred in schools where this prevention effort has been implemented" (1985a, p. 3). Barrett goes on to say that those who have evidence that suicide education in the schools increases the rate of suicide need to share their research.

Shaffer (1988) lists the following reasons why school-based curriculum programs need to be evaluated: Intuition is not a substitute for knowledge; the parts of the program that are effective need to be identified; and the concerns of parents, teachers, and administrators must be addressed and not just labeled as resistance. Shaffer stresses that we have a duty to evaluate suicide awareness programs, but the following problems are inherent in conducting such evaluations:

1. The suicide of a youth is rare and cannot be used as an outcome measure. This point has also been made by K. Smith (1988), who indi-

cates that a program must serve a large area and go on for many years before this type of evaluation becomes possible.

2. The easiest measure is how well the program is received; however, it is not entertainment but behavior change that we are after.

3. Attitude change can be measured before and after program participation, but most students have not experienced suicidal thoughts and may rate programs positively because of social expectancy factors.

4. Behavior measures such as actual intervention with a friend before versus after the program are more satisfactory.

5. Measures of suicide attempts before and after the program are needed. Increases after the program either could be the result of more awareness or could be caused by imitation factors.

Shaffer (1988) has called for a moratorium on curriculum presentations of suicide, and for extensive research in retrospect on those programs that have already been developed. Shaffer emphasizes that curriculum presentations are based on influencing decisions, and that most teen suicides are impulsive acts carried out while the youths are enraged, intoxicated, or in a state of terror. Many suicidal teens are therefore irrational and may not utilize resources and alternatives open to them.

K. Smith (1988) notes that one study showed that 9% of suicide attempters who had participated in a curriculum program felt that it made them worse, whereas 68% of attempters felt that the program helped them. Similarly, Shaffer (1988) notes that 91% of another group of attempters viewed a program as either positive or okay, whereas 9% rated the program negatively; the latter figure was statistically insignificant, but we still need to think about how to reach such youths. Shaffer also notes that attempters showed an increase in their preparedness to use crisis hotlines after program participation.

Shaffer (1988) recommends that more attention be paid to screening at-risk children. Instead of classroom presentations, efforts should concentrate on providing individual assistance to children at risk. Shaffer also recommends a number of activities for school personnel, such as training in the detection of suicidal students and promoting the availability of local hotlines and postvention programs. It seems clear that the one activity that Shaffer does not recommend is suicide awareness curriculum presentations.

Most school programs were originally developed because school personnel felt a need to do something. These programs began without much funding and most often without a research component, according to Ryerson (1988). Ryerson points out that as the number of programs grew and more students began to participate in curriculum units on suicide, researchers became interested in the effects of such programs. A collaborative effort between school program personnel and researchers is recommended by Ryerson.

There appears to be a consensus that it is important to evaluate the effectiveness of school programs, and I agree with that recommendation. I do feel that misinformation about suicide prevention is very common. A local administrator commented about a neighboring school district, "You know, once they developed a suicide prevention program, they started having suicides!" The administrator implied that it was best not to work on prevention; if one did, then somehow one created the behavior. The controversy about whether or not to have suicide awareness programs should not stop schools from having a suicide intervention program. Staff members need to be trained and procedures outlined. The components of such a program need to be clearly outlined to avoid generalizations and misconceptions.

Others have attempted to cite the increased demand for counseling by suicidal students as proof that these programs are not working. Ross (1985a) found that referrals to the counseling office increased 400% after a prevention program was implemented. Johnson and Maile (1987) indicate that referrals have tripled in some locations after a prevention program has been implemented. School counselors and school administrators need to recognize that an increase in the number of detected suicidal students and in the counseling services provided to them should be viewed positively. It means that the school system is doing a better job of detecting and providing service. It does *not* mean that having a school-based program causes suicidal behavior. It has been my personal experience that once students and staff are trained in detecting suicidal behavior, and once someone is identified as being willing and able to assist suicidal students, referrals will increase. I view the increased referrals positively and as an indication that our prevention efforts are working. It is important for schools to keep records of suicides, suicide attempts, referrals for counseling about suicidal thoughts, and the number of interventions by friends.

SUMMARY

The role of the schools is to detect suicidal behavior, assess the severity level of students' symptoms, notify parents, and secure the needed services for students. A crisis intervention model utilizing the three levels of intervention proposed by Caplan (1964) will help schools organize a comprehensive program. School staff members need training and confidence that they can make a difference in the problem of youth suicide. Schools need to follow up and assist students known to be suicidal.

Accurate records of interactions with suicidal students should be maintained, and evaluation procedures should be developed. Community resources to assist the schools should be identified, and a community-school partnership should be formed to work on this societal problem. The debate about whether or not suicide is an appropriate topic for a classroom discussion should never stop a school system from developing written guidelines to deal with suicidal students and providing training to school staff.

6

Liability and Legal Issues

A very real and practical question that school personnel need to ask concerns the responsibility and liability of the school system with regard to teenage suicide. Can a school system be sued for having an inadequate prevention program or no program at all? Can an individual employee be held liable either for acting improperly or for failing to act and provide assistance and supervision to a suicidal student? Is suicide a crime? Is it a crime to contribute to the suicide of another? These and many other questions have been raised about liability and legal issues for school personnel.

One of the few questions that has a simple answer is the question of whether or not suicide is a crime. Davidson (1985) reports that no states treat suicide as a crime. Two states, Oklahoma and Texas, list attempting suicide as a crime, but it is unlikely that the attempter will be prosecuted. Contributing to the suicide of another person by aiding his or her suicide attempt is a crime in 22 states, and individuals who have advised someone to commit suicide or who have helped them to obtain the instrument used to commit suicide have been prosecuted.

The California State Department of Education (1987) makes the following recommendation: "In light of potential legal actions, it is advisable for a school to provide student and staff training in teenage suicide prevention and to develop a suicide prevention policy" (p. 7). This very direct recommendation is the result of several lawsuits that have been filed against various school systems by the parents of students who have committed suicide. An examination of a few of those cases provides important insight into this issue.

WHEN ARE THE SCHOOLS LIABLE?:
AN EXAMINATION OF VARIOUS CASES

The issue of liability is not a new one. A Wisconsin school counselor was sued in 1960 for terminating counseling for a student who subsequently committed suicide. Davidson (1985) reports that the court found the counselor not liable because of no special training and no duty or control in the case. It seems logical that, given the dramatic rise in the youth suicide rate since 1960, counselors might be considered to have more responsibility today. Davidson cites cases going back as far as the 19th century in which surviving parents of suicide victims sought monetary damages against an individual or an institution. Davidson comments, "As a rule, the courts will not hold one person legally responsible for the suicide of another because suicide is considered a deliberate, intentional, intervening act. However, there are exceptions to this general rule" (1985, p. 300). Davidson cites three exceptions. The first one involves the intentional infliction of severe physical or emotional injury that leads someone to a suicidal state. An example of this would be the mother in Fort Lauderdale, Florida, who was found guilty in October 1987 of driving her teenage daughter to suicide. The mother was charged with child abuse and accused of forcing her daughter to become a nude dancer (*Houston Post*, January 22, 1988). A similar case involved an Illinois mother who sued her ex-husband for signing a gun permit, which enabled their son to obtain a gun that he used to commit suicide (*Houston Post*, September 21, 1987). This case has not been settled to date.

The second exception noted by Davidson (1985) is the violation of the law that prohibits the sale of liquor to a minor. There is no exception from liability when liquor is provided in violation of the law. I know of no court cases involving individuals who provided liquor to minors who committed suicide. I am somewhat surprised by this, in view of the frequency with which alcohol or drugs are consumed by teens shortly before committing suicide. It also seems likely that a person providing illegal drugs to a minor could be found liable if a suicide occurred while the minor was under the influence of those drugs.

The third exception discussed by Davidson is an institution's or a person's breach of legal duty to prevent a suicide. Davidson cites several cases where custodial care settings (e.g., jails, psychiatric hospitals, and reform schools) were found liable for not preventing the suicide of persons under their care. Henegar (1986) discusses liability issues with regard to runaway shelters and emphasizes that the primary issue is that of negligence. Henegar stresses the importance of duty of care and foreseeability of the actions of the client; he comments, "The legal issue is whether, based on knowledge known or expected to be known, the appropriate services were provided" (1986, p. 14). He also notes the importance of a full and detailed inquiry into the client's problems and into whether or not proper professional judgment was exercised. A major issue is whether or not the professional could have foreseen the suicidal risk of the client. Henegar comments, "It may help in understanding to realize that a negligence theory of liability in a suicide case is not generally a claim that one caused the suicide but rather that one did not take responsible steps to prevent that suicide (1986, p. 14). Henegar (1986) makes several recommendations to shelter personnel that have obvious implications for school personnel. Increased supervision of runaways (or students) should be provided, in combination with limiting their access to self-destructive instruments, and consideration should be given to getting additional psychological treatment for them.

Barrett (1985b) also discusses the issue of liability and school personnel, and concludes that the issue is unclear. In addition, Barrett discusses the question of whether an individual has the right to end his or her life without the interference or intervention of another person. He comments, "I believe that when it involves children, the ethical point has no meaning and suicide should always be prevented" (1985b, p. 45). This point is also stressed by Smith (1985), who emphasizes that those in the schools must intervene and not get caught in an ethical or philosophical dilemma about a teenager's right to end his or her life. I very strongly support this position. Barrett makes the following recommendations that should help school personnel avoid being found liable:

1. Make a referral to a more highly trained mental health specialist.
2. Seek supervision or collaboration on the case.
3. Know the ethics in your profession.
4. Keep records of your interactions with suicidal youth.

Several examples of liability issues in the schools are very interesting. A Denver teacher was put on leave after the suicide of one of her students. The teacher intercepted a note written by a 12-year-old seventh-grader and then read the very sensitive note aloud to the class. The student committed suicide later that day ("Teacher Put on Leave after Her Pupil's Suicide," 1987). At this writing, I do not know whether the teacher has been reinstated or whether a lawsuit has been filed.

One case that has received much attention and that has many implications for public school systems is the Kelson case from Oregon. Slenkovitch (1986) discusses this particular case, which involved a 14-year-old boy who committed suicide by shooting himself in the school restroom. The student, who was known to have a gun, was taken to the vice-principal's office after robbing a teacher of cash. The student gave the vice-principal a suicide note that he had written and requested to see his favorite teacher. The request was denied, and the police were called. The student shot himself while unsupervised in the restroom, after being told by the police that he was in serious trouble. The obvious questions to ask are those raised by Henegar: Was good professional judgment used, were the boy's actions foreseeable, was proper supervision provided, and were all lethal instruments removed? Unfortunately, it appears that the answers to each of these questions is no. Slenkovitch (1986) reports that the parents filed suit in federal court against the school. The federal district court dismissed the case, but the Ninth Circuit Court of Appeals found that the school was liable because the student's death resulted from the inadequate response of the school personnel and their lack of knowledge and preparation. Slenkovitch comments in part,

> The decision clearly opens the door to claims against the schools in cases of student suicide and even though the lawsuits may ultimately have no merit, the schools may be liable if a causal connection is found between a student's death or suicide attempt and an inadequate suicide prevention program. The obvious answer is to [provide] inservice [training for] staff. Never should staff take a suicide threat lightly. (1986, p. 3)

Slenkovitch (1986) also cautions against taking an authoritarian approach with suicidal students and recommends documentation of a "good-faith" effort on the part of the school system to prevent youth suicide.

Another case, in Milford, Connecticut, has implications for school systems. The parents of an eighth-grader filed suit against the Milford public school system following the suicide of their son at home. This was the first suit charging the school with responsibility for the actions of a student at a place other than at school (Johnson, 1987). The lawyer for the parents stressed that the school has an obligation to know when students are emotionally troubled and to notify the parents. This suit is still pending and has raised many questions about the responsibility of the schools versus the responsibility of the parents. Educators are concerned about where to draw the line with liability issues; they feel that the cost of liability insurance could skyrocket if the court finds in favor of these parents. The primary issue in the case is this: How accountable are the public schools when a student commits suicide? I am aware of other cases that raise similar questions.

HOW CAN SCHOOL PERSONNEL PROTECT THEMSELVES?

Hipple and Cimbolic (1979) stress the importance of mental health professionals' conducting themselves according to their professional standards and ethics. They note that malpractice suits are not based on making a wrong decision, but on gross negligence; negligence will be decided on the basis of foreseeability and control. Schutz (1982) states that it is important to ensure appropriate supervision for the suicidal student and not to withhold essential facts from parents. Mental health professionals in the schools are not expected to be perfect, and mistakes will occur. These mistakes will be examined on the basis of the information that the professionals have available to them.

The issue of the responsibility to warn parents has been at the basis of several lawsuits. Parents must be notified when a school staff member has any reason to believe that a youth is suicidal. This is at the basis of the school's liability protection and is clearly the appropriate action for school personnel to take. Whenever there is a concern about the welfare of a minor, the minor's parent or guardian must be notified. The challenge to the mental health professional in the schools is to make that notification in a manner that enlists parental support and increases supervision and services for the child. The questions of whether to report a suicidal child and whom to report the child to are among several issues addressed by Ruof et al. (1987), who consulted their school district's attorney. The following recommendations and conclusions from the attorney are helpful in several areas.

1. It is not sufficient to notify only the police. The parents of the suicidal youth must be notified. The attorney cited the *Tarasoff* doctrine, which addresses duty to warn.

2. School districts that have had suicides or suicidal threats should implement intervention programs.

3. The job description of mental health professionals in the schools should include working to assist suicidal youths, in order to cover the mental health professionals more clearly for insurance purposes.

4. School psychologists do have greater responsibility than other employees to take action to assist suicidal youths, and must follow professional ethics. Suicidal students can and should be seen with or without parent permission.

5. School personnel who have responsibility for a child (bus drivers, teachers, etc.) should be advised if a student is suicidal, so that appropriate supervision can be provided.

These recommendations are very straightforward, and I support each of them. School psychologists need to recognize their increased liability and take leadership roles in this area. Their job description should include working with suicidal students. I recommend seeing the student first and then notifying the parents. Several states have passed legislation that allow treatment of a minor by a mental health professional without parental consent.

As noted earlier (see Chapter 5, "Parent Notification"), the state of Texas passed Senate Bill 1122 in 1985; this legislation allows physicians, psychologists, counselors, and social workers to provide services to a minor without parental consent under certain circumstances (situations involving sexual abuse, physical abuse, or suicide prevention). Other states besides Texas may have similar legislation. Assistance can and should be provided to a suicidal student with or without parental consent, but it is essential that the *parents be notified* that their child is believed to be suicidal. Childress (1985), in discussing this type of legislation, points out that adults have always been free to refuse medical or psychological help for themselves, but that they cannot use their views as a basis for withholding needed help for their children. Courts recognize parents' rights, but not at the expense of children's not getting the help that they need. Childress (1985) and Barrett (1985b) both speculated that mandatory reporting laws for suicidal behavior in children may be in place in the near future.

Texas Senate Bill 1122 also addresses the question of liability for mental health professionals. The law states that these professionals are not liable for civil damages when they treat suicidal youths unless they engage in willful misconduct or gross negligence. The question of the liability of school employees is also addressed as part of the Wisconsin Youth Suicide Prevention Act, which was passed in 1985. The legislation contains a civil liability exemption for school employees (Wisconsin Department of Instruction, 1986). The exemption states,

> Any school board, private school, county handicapped children's education board or cooperative educational service agency and any officer employee or volunteer thereof, who in good faith attempts to prevent suicide by a pupil is immune from civil liability for his or her acts or omissions in respect to the suicide or attempted suicide. (quoted by Wisconsin Department of Instruction, 1986, p. 112)

Omissions that might expose a school employee to liability as not having acted in "good faith" are undoubtedly failures in the areas of duty to care, duty to warn, and foreseeability.

SUMMARY AND RECOMMENDATIONS

It is clear that there is much uncertainty in the areas of legality and liability with regard to youth suicide. Numerous court cases are pending, and some school administrators have elected to do nothing in the way of establishing a formal prevention program because of their uncertainty about the responsibility of the school. It appears clear to me that schools are increasingly being found liable for not taking action to work on this societal problem. One administrator remarked to me that the schools have to be willing to face the problem and take some risk to establish an intervention program. Similarly, Johnson and Maile (1987) comment that "the problem is inescapable and so is the responsibility" (p. 1). I agree completely with their assessment, and I recommend that school systems establish programs using the following guidelines:

1. A written policy should outline prevention, intervention, and post-vention activities, and this policy should be updated every 2 years.

2. Legal counsel should be sought in developing guidelines.

3. All school personnel should receive in-service training on how to detect suicidal behavior and should understand the referral procedures. There should be a brief annual in-service update on warning signs.

4. Identified mental health specialists in the school system should be familiar with the ethics of their particular professions and should receive intensive training on working with suicidal youths; their job description should delineate their role in working with suicidal students.

5. The parents of a suicidal youth must be notified.

6. Suicidal youths should be supervised closely, and any lethal instruments should be kept away from them.

7. Community resources should be identified to assist suicidal youths.

8. Suicidal youths should be monitored and assisted as long as they attend the school system.

9. Complete and accurate records should be maintained on all suicidal youths.

10. All school personnel who work directly with a suicidal student should be notified that the student is suicidal.

11. School mental health specialists should collaborate on cases of suicidal youths and should refer to mental health specialists outside of the schools.

12. School employees should be familiar with state and national legislation concerning their professions and the area of suicide prevention.

13. The school mental health specialists should ask detailed and comprehensive questions about a student's history, family history, and plans to commit suicide.

14. The school system should assume an active role in working on this problem and should coordinate intervention efforts with all appropriate area agencies.

7

Legislation

There has been growing awareness at the federal level that youth suicide is a mental health problem that our nation must face. Numerous bills have been introduced at the national level to address the problem. Representative Gary Ackerman from New York has commented, "Any loss of life is tragic. The loss of a child is devastating. The self-inflicted death of a youngster is an unthinkable horror. Yet think we must so that we can understand and prevent it" (quoted by Landis, 1987a, p. 3). There has been much discussion of what can be done at the national level, and some things have been done. This chapter describes the national legislative efforts and also discusses individual states' legislative efforts. Several states have passed legislation concerning youth suicide prevention. What that legislation means for the schools and what the trend may be for the future will be outlined. Texas has now passed a resolution concerning youth suicide. I was active in drafting that resolution and testified in favor of it to members of the state legislature.

EFFORTS AT THE NATIONAL LEVEL

A National Conference on Youth Suicide was held in Washington, D.C., in June 1985. The conference was cosponsored by the U.S. Department of Health and Human Services and the Youth Suicide National Center. The objectives of the conference were to raise public awareness, disseminate information, undertake research, and demonstrate services to help with the problem of youth suicide (Farberow, Altman, & Thorne, 1985). The conference brought 500 nationally recognized professionals in the field together to explain the problem and inform the nation. President Reagan signed into law a resolution designating June 1985 as "Youth Suicide Prevention Month." Charlotte Ross (1985c) has commented on the conference,

> In many ways, it was a historic occasion, one that confirmed that we are prepared as a nation to face a large problem whose solution was not easy. No society, including ours, likes to take on a condition that is not only complicated, but traditionally considered shameful, sinful and embarrassing or even criminal. This conference said clearly that avoidance and denial are no longer acceptable alternatives. (p. xxi)

Ross notes that youth suicide was declared an epidemic by the World Health Organization in the 1970s and that efforts to work on the epidemic up until the 1980s were largely undertaken at the community level. One of the early national efforts was a grant provided by the Department of Health and Human Services to produce suicide prevention training materials for runaway shelter personnel.

Government hearings on this topic were first held by the House of Representatives Select Committee on Children, Youth and Families in 1983, according to Harris and Crawford (1987). The first federal bill addressing youth suicide was introduced in the U.S. Congress in 1984. President Reagan commented in part that "suicide is no longer a silent subject but a recognized public health problem that can and must be addressed" (quoted by Ross, 1985c, p. xxv). Reagan emphasized the responsibility and opportunity that all citizens have to work on this problem.

The Youth Suicide National Center was established in 1985. It is a nonprofit organization that receives donations from the private sector. Charlotte Ross is the executive director of the center, which has offices in Washington, D.C., and Burlingame, California. Ross (1985b) emphasizes that the purpose of the center is to serve as a source of information, guidance, and leadership to support and improve prevention efforts. She notes the need to bring the problem to the attention of the public and to work with the government on various levels. The center provides support for self-help groups at the local and regional level, disseminates information about state legislations, and encourages the formation of survivor groups and the creation of crisis hotlines.

Margaret Heckler, Secretary of the U.S. Department of Health and Human Services, established the department's Task Force of Youth Suicide Prevention in 1985; this task force has held three meetings to date. It has concentrated on compiling information on risk factors and intervention programs, and is working on recommendations for research and education services. In addition (as noted in earlier chapters), the OIG, a division of the Department of Health and Human Services, was asked to conduct a national program inspection of youth suicide to supplement the work done by the task force. This inspection involved surveying 348 experts in the field, and more than half the respondents recommended that the federal government assume a more active role through supporting research, establishing national policies to support youths and the family, and providing funding for suicide prevention programs (OIG, 1986).

The National Association of School Psychologists, the American Association of Counselor Development, and the AAS have all actively supported federal legislative efforts in this area. Each organization has legislative officers and committees working with interested senators and representatives. Professionals are encouraged to contact their respective professional organizations to keep up with legislative developments.

Harris and Crawford (1987) reported that the Youth Suicide Prevention Act passed the U.S. House of Representatives in June 1986 and was referred to the Senate Subcommittee on Education. The bill would have established grants to provide funds to establish and operate prevention programs, both in the schools and at private nonprofit organizations. Harris and Crawford have emphasized the important role assigned to school counselors in this legislation, as well as the requirement of evaluation procedures for prevention programs.

House of Representatives Bill 457 (H.R. 457) was sponsored by Representative Ackerman from New York and Representative Lantos of California and introduced in 1987. This legislation would provide $1 million to increase awareness of youth suicide, to train school and community leaders, and to coordinate prevention efforts. Lantos commented in part, "We are looking at a national tragedy that demands a national response and H.R. 457 is a critical first step" (quoted by Landis, 1987a, p. 1). I have written to the Youth Suicide National Center to find out the fate of the Youth Suicide Prevention Act and the House of Representatives Bill 457, but have not received a response.

A similar bill was introduced in the Senate by Senator Lautenberg of New Jersey. Senate Bill 1199 would provide several million dollars each year from 1988 to 1991 to fund demonstration projects, to establish prevention programs to work on the problem, and to conduct research in the area of youth suicide. The most recent information that I have on the status of this bill is from the Youth Suicide National Center, which reported that the bill was read twice and referred to the Committee on Labor and Human Resources.

No federal legislation has passed to date, and it is difficult to explain why. Phyllis Schafly, as previously mentioned, has been very outspoken against "death education," and other extreme conservatives also appear not to support suicide prevention legislation. Schafly (1985) has cited numerous examples of school curricula that have forced teenagers to deal with depressing themes. She comments, "I believe it is clear that any real attempt to prevent teenage suicide must start with an expose of the suicide promoting materials they are given in class and the rock music lyrics they listen to" (1985, p. 274). Schafly has further stressed that teenage suicide is exactly why the 1978 Pupil Protection Amendment was necessary:

> It is clear that the psychological death and suicide courses described in the hearings were given to children without prior parental consent. Teachers must be prohibited from playing amateur psychologist or psychiatrist or therapist without a license while imposing experimental treatment on normal, healthy children. (1985, p. 274)

The 1978 Pupil Protection Amendment (also known as the Hatch Amendment) requires that parents give written consent prior to their child's participating in experimental psychological programs. Davis et al. (1988) state that school personnel should be made aware of this amendment in regard to the screening of suicidal students.

Schafly's objections to suicide prevention programs clearly fall in the area of curriculum and presentations to students that deal directly with the topic of suicide. I disagree with her position, but do see a reason why debate could arise about the advisability of such a direct approach. What I cannot understand is why conservatives do not support the proposed national legislation, which emphasizes in-service training for school personnel in detecting suicidal behavior and in assisting suicidal students. The legislation does not emphasize or even directly mention suicide as a curriculum topic. It appears that misperceptions about youth suicide exist, along with denial about the extent of the problem and confusion about whose responsibility it is to work on the problem.

EFFORTS IN INDIVIDUAL STATES

Several states have passed legislation having to do with youth suicide prevention. Each state has taken a slightly different approach. I have been most active with supporting the legislation in Texas, but I also serve on the School Legislative Subcommittee of the AAS, which supports efforts in several states.

California

The first state that passed legislation in this area was California in 1983. Senate Bill 947 contained a long-range plan to reduce youth suicide in California. This legislation provided a 3-year pilot project to develop guidelines for a statewide program. O'Connor (1985) has described the California State Department of Education's close work in the first year of the project with two programs, one of which was in the Los Angeles area and the other in the San Francisco area. These school programs had received much guidance from the crisis centers located in those cities. The role of the state department of education was to set broad criteria for the programs and to provide adequate funding so that school districts could have greater flexibility and could utilize local resources.

The second year of the project concentrated efforts on workshops that reached personnel from over 250 schools. The role of parents, teachers, and students was emphasized in prevention efforts. Harris and Crawford (1987) note that the model allowed for both an in-school classroom approach and a non-classroom-based approach utilizing community resources. An examination of Senate Bill 947 shows objectives that fall into several levels of intervention, including enhancement of the school climate, improved decision making, understanding of the relationship of drugs and alcohol to suicide, student knowledge of community resources such as hotlines, accurate data collection, parent and teacher training, and postvention procedures.

Peck (1985) notes that a curriculum was developed in the third year of the project that contained five classroom sessions for students, emphasizing understanding and coping with depression and how to respond to a suicidal friend. The curriculum was appropriate for use in several classes. The role of the teacher and the importance of detecting suicidal students were also stressed. Peck has also emphasized the importance of evaluating the results of such a curriculum approach to see whether students were helped by it. The legislation required that an evaluation of the project as a whole be submitted to the governor by January 1987.

As noted above, the ultimate goal of Senate Bill 947 was to develop a statewide prevention program, and $300,000 in funding for such a program was provided. It was stressed that a priority for funding was to support those existing programs that were successful. The department of education was charged with reporting to the legislature on progress in this area annually. The California approach is a very comprehensive one, emphasizing the importance of having programs at the primary, secondary, and tertiary crisis intervention levels. There are few data available at this writing on the effectiveness of the program. The California State

Department of Education (1987) has published a book entitled *Suicide Prevention Program for the California Public Schools.*

New Jersey

The state of New Jersey passed legislation in 1985 that created youth suicide prevention programs in three regions of the state and created a Youth Suicide Prevention Advisory Council. Richard Codey, Chairman of the Senate Committee on Institutions, Health and Welfare, introduced this legislation by stating, "If suicide were a disease, we'd be spending millions to find the cause and treat it" (quoted by Dunne-Maxim, 1985, p. 183). Dunne-Maxim (1985) notes that legislative hearings provided the opportunity for many suicide survivors and mental health professionals to testify in favor of the legislation. The bill provides $300,000 in funding. The bill established objectives in several areas: classroom instruction to teach the warning signs of suicide to students; training school personnel to detect suicidal students; programs to educate parents; improved linkage with community programs; and provision of assistance to the families of survivors. The pilot program will be evaluated and a report submitted to the governor. Suicide awareness materials have been developed and distributed throughout the state.

Wisconsin

In 1985, Wisconsin passed legislation that emphasized coordination of prevention efforts throughout the state. There were several major objectives. A Youth Suicide Prevention Council was created, with representatives from the state departments of education, mental health, and criminal justice. Each of 12 cooperative educational agencies across the state received $3,000 in funding. Training programs in suicide prevention were required in both the public and private schools. School districts were given until July 1988 to have a suicide prevention curriculum in place. The legislation protected from liability anyone acting in good faith who referred a student for being suicidal.

The Wisconsin Department of Instruction (1986) has published a book entitled *Suicide Prevention: A Resource and Planning Guide.* This publication states that the objectives of the 1985 legislation were to increase awareness of suicidal behavior and to create a curriculum to deal with suicide prevention. The curriculum places emphasis on decision making, knowledge of conditions that contribute to suicide, the warning signs, the relationship of drugs and alcohol to suicide, knowledge of community resources, and positive emotional development for students.

Florida

Florida passed legislation in 1984 that required a coordinated effort among state agencies to develop a plan for youth suicide prevention. The title of the legislation was The Florida Youth Emotional Development and Suicide Prevention Act. A plan was accordingly submitted by the Florida Department of Health and Human Services to the governor. As McKinney (1985) describes it, the plan was for each of 11 health and rehabilitation service districts throughout the state to develop a continuum of services that included prevention, public awareness, peer counseling, community- and agency-coordinated education, and training for parents and school staff. Intervention efforts through hotlines and crisis agencies and shelters were included, as were treatment services such as emergency room services and hospitalization for suicidal youths. Funding recommendations were part of the state plan. McKinney notes that although the plan was sent to the governor, it was not introduced before the state legislature.

The Florida approach has received some criticism, and the lack of funding from the legislature has resulted in very little being implemented. Harris and Crawford (1987) state,

> First, Florida's helping professionals have been expected to finance their crisis intervention program with existing strained resources. Second, district reports of available services and assessments of local situations were drafted too rapidly resulting in an inadequate state report. Finally, the various departments involved in the provision of services—education, law enforcement, health and rehabilitation—appear to be unclear regarding their individual responsibilities. (p. 52)

Harris and Crawford also note that the testimony of two parent advocate groups resulted in a requirement of parental permission for a student to be exposed to suicide prevention programs. Perhaps the state overreacted to the concerns of the parent groups.

Alabama

Alabama passed legislation in 1985 emphasizing the need for cooperation among numerous agencies to work on prevention. A task force was created, and local districts were instructed to develop a plan of action. Harris and Crawford (1987) note the comprehensive nature of the services to be made available to school children. Each school must have a written plan of student services, including suicide awareness. The Alabama Youth Education Guidance and Suicide Prevention Act also examined life management or wellness as a curriculum topic early in high school, and required that teachers be able to recognize the warning signs of suicide.

Texas

I was contacted in 1987 by a Texas state representative, Frank Collazo, and invited to assist with the drafting of legislation in regard to youth suicide. I met with him and a committee of professionals on several occasions. A very basic question that arose was this: "Who is qualified to train school personnel in the area of suicide prevention? The committee and I felt that the wording of this in the legislation should be fairly general, specifying only that training should be done by someone who has demonstrated knowledge and has had experience in this area. We did not feel that the legislation should specify that training could only be done by psychologists, social workers, counselors, or certified crisis center personnel. We knew that much of Texas is rural, and that small school districts may not have any such professionals on staff or even nearby.

We surveyed other states and examined their legislation, and made a number of recommendations that comprised House Bill 1631. The bill would have required the Texas Education Agency to develop training materials for school staff, including written policies and procedures, a service directory for referrals, procedures for identifying at-risk students, models for cooperation among the schools and various state and private agencies, procedures for assisting students identified as suicidal, procedures for postvention, and media guidelines. Annual in-service training for school personnel on suicide prevention was to be required. Three other professionals and I testified in support of this legislation before the House Committee on Public Education.

Our testimony was not received as well as we had hoped for. I will not go into specifics here, but suicide prevention is a topic on which many misperceptions and much denial exist. The chairman of the committee was very abrupt with his comments, and it was difficult to say all that we wanted to on the topic. There was no stated opposition; in fact, several groups such as the state PTA and teachers' associations voiced their support. We did not have any parents who had survived the suicide of a child testify, and perhaps that would have made more of an impact. This bill was then put in the hands of a subcommittee; thanks to the tireless efforts of Representative Collazo, a resolution did pass and was signed by the governor in June 1987.

I learned a great deal through participating in this process. One of the things that I learned is that a bill passed by the state legislature *requires* something, and a resolution merely *recommends* that something be done.

House Resolution 168 directs the Texas Education Agency to study the causes and factors related to youth suicide. This study will include examining the curriculum at all grade levels with regard to such areas as decision making, problem solving, self-esteem, wellness life styles, and coping with emotions. The agency will report its curriculum findings to the legislature, along with recommendations for in-service training for school personnel. There has been discussion of the possibility that the agency would provide resources to school districts and perhaps even a designated suicide expert to travel to school districts to provide training and intervention. This resolution is not all that I would like, but it is a start. I am presently serving on the State Task Force on Youth Suicide Prevention, which has been created by the Texas Education Agency.

Two other state legislators have contacted me about their ideas for legislation that would address the problem of youth suicide from a more comprehensive viewpoint, which would involve state mental health and law enforcement agencies. These legislators are in the initial stages of gathering information.

SUMMARY AND CONCLUSIONS

It is difficult to predict whether or not legislation on suicide intervention will be passed at the national level. It is needed to support existing programming efforts, to implement more intervention programs, and to fund research that would provide invaluable guidance to all who are working on this societal problem. It is encouraging that several states have passed legislation. There is much that can be done, but how to do it is a very complex question. A carefully planned approach, to be carried out in several steps over a period of years and adequately funded, would seem to be ideal. Almost every state has done something; those states that have not introduced legislation have at least formed committees to examine the severity of the problem and begin communication about it. According to the OIG (1986), 35 states had addressed youth suicide in some way as of 1986.

An examination of what individual states have done in this area shows many differences. Some of the legislation is very vague, especially about what is required of an individual school district. A school district should be allowed to use its resources and those in the community to address this problem in a productive way, but should not be allowed to pretend that the problem of youth suicide does not exist. It is also important to recognize that problems that young people have, such as drug and alcohol abuse, conduct problems, and suicidal tendencies, are inextricably linked and all need addressing.

8

The School and Postvention

"Few events in a school are more painful or potentially more disruptive than the suicide of a student" (Lamb & Dunne-Maxim, 1987, p. 245). A suicide touches everyone, and the school community itself becomes a survivor of suicide. It has been estimated that a suicide results in a 300% increase in the likelihood that others at the school will commit suicide (Lamartine, 1985). The one question that school personnel are probably the least trained to deal with and the most apprehensive about is what to do in the immediate aftermath of a suicide. Many times nothing is done, and experts have cautioned that doing nothing is dangerous (Boggs, 1987; Lamb & Dunne-Maxim, 1987). Kneisel and Richards (1988) point out that a distinction must be made between responses that increase the size of the affected community and those that help individuals who will learn of the event. They stress that postvention gives the schools the chance to improve prevention efforts. Students at school will learn of the event and need an opportunity to talk about it.

The term "postvention" is one with which school personnel may not be very familiar. Shneidman (1985) describes the process of working with the bereaved after a suicide as "postvention," with the purpose being to help survivors live longer, more productive, and less stressful lives. A number of steps that can be taken after a suicide to minimize the contagion effects and maximize the preventive effects (Lamb & Dunne-Maxim, 1987).

Although Hill (1984) notes that little information is available to guide school systems after a suicide, two suicidologists (Biblarz, 1988; Ryerson, 1988) have emphasized that the question is not whether there should be talk about the suicide, but instead how to talk about it. They stress that an emotionally neutral presentation should give students the facts that they need to know. However, many other questions have been raised.

Should a large assembly be held to discuss the suicide with other students? Who should direct the postvention efforts, and is an outside consultant needed? Should the family of the deceased be contacted? These and other questions are addressed in this chapter to guide the schools in postvention. The incidence of youth suicide indicates that most school systems will be faced at some point with a postvention situation. Postvention provides the opportunity to get administrative support for suicide intervention programs. As noted earlier, most school-based programs are developed in response to a previous tragedy.

I have been involved in numerous postvention situations; each one was slightly different, but many common themes were evident, and the basic approach that is recommended is the same. Two case examples may help illustrate this process.

CASE STUDY 1

An 18-year-old high school boy, L, made numerous suicidal threats over the course of a few days. He stated to his peers, "I won't be at the party Saturday. I'll be in hell by then! Here's my class ring; I won't need it any more." He asked several questions of friends: "Why is life worth living? What would it be like if your friend was suddenly dead and you never saw him again? What would it feel like to hang yourself with a rope? What is there to live for? We are all going to die anyway. Would you like my car? I am going to give it away." These were very definite clues of suicidal behavior. Unfortunately, none of the friends of the young man detected these signals and notified an adult.

L was also using drugs heavily over the course of the days leading up to his suicide. On at least one school day, he was too depressed to come into the school building and spent much of the day sitting alone in his car in the parking lot. Several of his teachers were concerned about his behavior. One later commented,

> He didn't seem himself; he was depressed and lethargic. I tried to get him to talk with me, but he wouldn't. I asked him what was wrong, but he wouldn't answer. That very day that he hung himself, I had asked him to come and talk with me after school, but he didn't. I feel terrible about this. I should have somehow done more. He didn't say anything about suicide, but he did seem very depressed.

On the day he died, L went home from school at the regular time. No one was home, and he hanged himself. His father was worried about him and had been waiting to talk with him, but had left to run to the store for a few things. Afterward, the father commented,

> I knew that he was under a lot of stress with school, work, and all. He had failed a couple of classes and had written a bad check to pay for work on his car. I've been married a bunch of times and I am an alcoholic, and we have had our share of problems. I haven't been there when he needed me. I almost went into his room the night before to wake him up to talk with him. I wanted to tell him that things would get better and that I would help him. I just didn't think things were that bad. I never thought that he would kill himself. Do you think that if I had talked with him, he might not have done this? I was waiting that afternoon to talk with him. I just left for a few minutes. When I came back and saw his car in the driveway, I thought, "Good, we will get a chance to talk, just the two of us." I went in and found him dead. Later, I found the suicide note that he had taped to the mirror of his room. I don't know how long it had been there. He didn't blame anybody. The note said it was just too painful to live any more. I also found a list that he had made of all his relatives; he was checking them off as he saw them all for the last time. I don't know how I am going to get through this. He's gone!

A number of postvention steps were taken at suicide to minimize the impact of the suicide. A summary of those steps appears below:

1. A calling tree was used to alert key faculty members.

2. A faculty meeting was held before school to give the faculty the facts and to allow them to express their emotions.

3. A counselor followed L's schedule and attended his classes to help the students and faculty cope with his death. Students in his class were given the opportunity to express their emotions in writing. Students were also involved in the process of deciding what to do with L's chair in each classroom.

4. A counselor and psychologist made contact with his family and offered assistance.

5. The death was honestly acknowledged and discussed in a home-room format, rather than in a large assembly. Students were given information on how to detect suicidal behavior and what to do to get help if they detected suicidal behavior. The local crisis hotline number was posted in all classrooms.

6. Counselors and psychologists began networking efforts. The networking involved two groups of students: those previously known to have been suicidal, and those who were close to L.

7. The teacher who had been most concerned about L was given individual counseling.

8. A spokesperson was designated to meet with media representatives.

9. The superintendent's office was kept informed.

10. A support group was held for troubled parents at school in the evening.

11. It was suggested to the family that the funeral be on the following Saturday, rather than on a school day.

12. All school activities were continued, and grieving students were encouraged to participate as much as possible in normal activities.

13. L had a younger sister in grade school, and her counselor was immediately notified so that support could be offered to her.

14. A request to dedicate a school dance to L was later denied; instead, students were encouraged to donate money to the library in his name.

A couple of unique points about this postvention case stand out in my mind. I particularly remember the counselors at the school commenting, "We know what to do; we have been through this before; and we have confidence that we can assist all concerned." No media attention was paid to this particular suicide; one isolated teen suicide in a large metropolitan area is not news. No students at the school attempted suicide in the next few days or weeks.

The suicide of L had a profound effect on his friends and his neighborhood, but not on the school of 2,500 as a whole, because he was not known to a large segment of the student body. His friends were devastated by his suicide. Many had known him for years and had gone through many years of school with him. Those students who had been given direct suicidal clues were especially guilt-ridden and asked many difficult questions, such as "If I had told someone what he said about death, do you think that he would still be alive?" Questions like these are very difficult to answer. My answer was "We cannot be sure, but he might still be alive." It is important that students know about the situational nature of suicide for the future. These students needed much emotional support to deal with the loss of their friend and the guilt that they felt. I also stressed that L was the only person who was responsible for his actions. Several students were referred to outside practitioners for more in-depth assistance.

A number of parents from the community called or came to the school for conferences. They asked many questions about youth suicide and were greatly troubled by L's suicide. There were a couple of common themes to their comments. First, they couldn't believe what had happened. One mother commented, "L had breakfast at my house that morning. He seemed okay. How could he do this?" A second theme was how they could help their children cope with this. A father stated, "My son won't talk with me about it. This is the worst thing that has ever happened to him. I want to help him, but I don't know how."

It was decided after a number of such parent conferences to hold a support group at the school for parents. It was felt that there was a need for a meeting, and it would be better for the high school to volunteer to have such a meeting instead of waiting for parents to demand one. The principal, the counselors, and I all had some trepidation about conducting such a meeting, but decided to go ahead. All the parents of L's friends were called and invited to an evening meeting. Many of the parents who were invited expressed appreciation. A counselor called me in somewhat of a panic and said that L's father had heard about the meeting and wanted to attend; what did I think about that? I knew that his attendance would intensify the meeting, but I also felt that he had a right to attend. In addition, he was certainly in need of support and might not receive it anywhere else. He attended, along with L's stepmother.

The meeting was attended by approximately 25 parents, all but two of whom had known L. One of L's friends also attended. The meeting was held in the home economics suite to provide a more comfortable setting. I directed the meeting and made a few introductory statements. I let the group know that I was a survivor of a suicide, and this heightened my credibility. It was very apparent that L's father had a need to talk, and he described the sequence of events that led up to his son's suicide. He also disclosed much about his personal life. His wife was relatively quiet. The most difficult point was when the father asked, "Would he still be alive if I had talked with him the night before he died?" I answered that in the most tactful and supportive way that I could: "We cannot know for sure, but suicidal young people do not truly want to die, and can be and have been helped." I also told the father about the local survivors' group and recommended that he become involved in their meetings.

A parent who had not known L personally then introduced herself and stated that she had known several other young people who had committed suicide. She was angry about this and felt that such deaths would not occur if parents loved and cared for their children. This translated into an attack on L's parents and was responded to immediately by L's stepmother. The two counselors and I spent the next 30 minutes processing these statements and supporting L's parents. The focus was then shifted to what could be done to help L's friends, and general information on youth suicide was shared. The friend who was present spoke up and said that his parents had made him come to the meeting and that he had resented it; however, he stressed that he had learned a lot and that he would share it with L's other friends. He knew that the parents cared and wanted to communicate with their children and to help them through this. He stated, "Communication between parents and teenagers is the key to solving the problem of youth suicide, and if L had told his parents how bad things were, he'd be alive today." I agreed with him about the importance of communication, and after more discussion, the meeting was adjourned.

Several parents stayed for a few minutes of individual help. I privately thanked L's parents for attending and stressed the importance of becoming involved with the survivors' group. The counselors and I stayed to process the meeting with one another and to provide support for one another. Several parents called or sent notes thanking the school for its extra efforts to help with the problem of youth suicide. The principal was very pleased that the meeting had gone well. Follow-up counseling was provided to the students who needed it, especially to L's younger sister. I called L's parents on several occasions and reminded them of my recommendation that they attend the survivors' support group. They always seemed interested, but never attended a meeting.

CASE STUDY 2

One of our high schools experienced two suicides within a 6-week period. The aftermath of these two suicides was very traumatic for the school and the community. A number of postvention steps were taken and are outlined here.

I was notified at 8 A.M. of the suicide of a 10th-grade boy, G, the night before by carbon monoxide poisoning. Upon my arrival on the campus, the principal convened his administrative and counseling team. He announced the suicide and then indicated that I would direct the postvention efforts. This high school had not previously experienced a suicide; however, it had a very well-trained crisis team that had responded admirably to other student deaths.

One issue that surfaced immediately was the question of whether the death was a suicide or an accident. One staff member offered the thought that perhaps the student had fallen asleep listening to the radio in the garage. A discussion followed that perhaps we should announce the death as an accident. I thought otherwise and was very emphatic that we get the facts and deal with the death honestly and openly. The principal and I agreed to go to the home and talk directly with the parents to verify the circumstances surrounding the death, to express our condolences, and to offer assistance to the family—particularly to the surviving ninth-grade brother. I am all for reaching out to the families of suicide victims, but I was nervous as we approached the home. The parents recognized the principal immediately and welcomed our visit. We were told that the death was indeed a suicide, and the parents were very cooperative and interested in our plans to assist the students at school. We introduced ourselves to the younger brother and offered support. We discussed funeral arrangements and formed a relationship with the family that was very positive and close and that continues to this day.

The principal and I returned to school and clarified that the death was a suicide. A memorandum to all faculty was immediately sent out, with specific information about the warning signs of suicide and guidelines for dealing with a crisis. Teachers were encouraged to model the expression of feelings and to let students discuss their feelings. The memorandum encouraged teachers to send those students who were most upset to the counselors' office. A counselor and a psychologist followed G's class schedule and spoke to his classmates.

Students asked such questions as these: "How did he do it? Why did he do it? How is his brother doing? Did his friends know what he was planning? Do you think he is in hell? Why didn't God stop him? What should you do if a friend talks about suicide? When is the funeral? Did he suffer? How long did it take him to die? Did he use drugs?" Our strategy was to honestly acknowledge the death by suicide, but to downplay the method and the questions about why G committed suicide. I emphasized that the reasons why G committed suicide would never be known for sure, because the information had died with him. I stressed that we were here to help the students cope and that the focus was on them, their reactions, and their future. We talked extensively about intervention by friends and the situational nature of suicide. Many students were in a state of shock.

Other postvention procedures discussed in the first case example were utilized, such as making a list of students believed to be at risk and conducting a faculty meeting. I also talked with the driver of G's bus about what to say to students that afternoon. Phone contact was made with the family, and arrangements were made to ease the re-entry of the younger brother to school. I talked with him prior to his return and talked to each of his teachers about how to handle his return to school.

Many parents called and asked questions about reaching out to the family, funeral attendance, and issues concerning their own children. The counseling staff stayed very focused on grief resolution and suicide prevention for several weeks. A number of school personnel attended the funeral. The service was conducted by a family member who was a minister, and it was a beautiful combination of religion and mental health. The minister acknowledged that G had had problems and identified them. Teenagers were encouraged not to do what G had done, and the uniqueness of his problems and the situational nature of suicidal thoughts were stressed. The minister addressed the question of why God didn't stop G. The minister said that God had sounded an alarm, but God couldn't stop him. God embraced G, yes, but felt robbed of many years on earth in which G could have done his work. The service itself, and its message to the surviving classmates and friends, were very preventive. Counseling services have been provided to the surviving brother, and close contact with the brother and the family will, I am sure, continue until the younger brother graduates.

The second suicide occurred 6 weeks later. A ninth-grade girl, S, who had known G only slightly, shot herself at home. Much the same postvention steps were taken as in G's case. The general mood of the counseling and administrative team was one of calmness, competence, and sadness. The family was contacted immediately, and two counselors went to the home. The girl had an 11th-grade sister who attended the same high school. Many students were quickly identified as upset, and several counselors and psychologists were called in from their assignments at other schools.

S was identified as someone who was known to be at risk. Her parents had been notified, and private psychological and psychiatric services had been provided to her. The administrative question was asked: Had the school done everything possible to prevent this suicide? There was a slight undercurrent of placing blame. I addressed this question directly. The school had previously detected the girl as suicidal, notified parents, secured more services, and followed up and monitored her progress. I stated that we had done all we could; it was a sad situation, but no one was to blame. There are a few adolescents who follow through and kill themselves despite professional intervention.

About 15 of S's friends were not in school; they had gathered to grieve at one of their houses. A parent of one student called and asked what to do to help them. I suggested that the students come to school so that counselors and psychologists could work with them. They came to school, stayed about an hour, and were dealt with as a group. Because they felt out of place at school, two counselors accompanied them to one of their homes, where a minister joined them. The group processing helped everyone. A teacher made a positive comment the next day about how this group of students was coping.

One student who came to the counseling office immediately for assistance was the younger brother of G. He had become quite upset as soon as he heard about the second suicide. I called his parents and notified them of what had happened. He talked with them, and that helped him calm down. He and his parents expressed the wish to reach out and support S's family. I agreed to call S's family and to convey their offer of assistance. The members of S's family were very receptive to that idea, and G's family visited them that very evening.

Counselors and psychologists visited each of S's classes and led a discussion with students. This went well in all but one class. We had visited this teacher's class 6 weeks previously, after the first suicide. The teacher knew why we were there and immediately said, "Do you want to talk to the students before or after they take their test?" I was appalled by the mention of a test on this day. I looked around the room and saw three students crying, one of whom was the younger brother of G, whom I had just finished consoling. I recommended that there be no test that day. The teacher responded that there had to be a test to keep up with the rest of the teaching team and to avoid having to make a separate form of the test for those students. I firmly repeated my statement, which was supported by the school counselor. The teacher disappeared; she came back after checking with the team leader and reluctantly agreed to postpone the test. A central issue is that in postvention, academic plans, particularly tests, may have to be altered. I recommend that the administrative memorandum giving teachers the facts about the suicide also spell out that the curriculum may have to be set aside in certain classes. A student in another of S's classes raised his hand and stated that we must be worried about contagion. I answered this by stating that S had her unique problems, noting that suicidal thoughts were situational, and emphasizing alternatives.

The high school decided to publicize the local crisis hotline and the importance of friend intervention. We developed the card shown in Figure 8.1, which was printed by the media department in record time. Each of the 2,500 students in the high school was given a billfold-sized version of this card, and a larger one was posted in each classroom. The student body president discussed the card and suicide prevention during morning announcements. The president did a superb job and commented, "If your friend was hurt in an accident, you would take them to a doctor! If your friend is hurting inside, get adult help for him!"

DON'T KEEP A SECRET - SAVE A LIFE by telling your parents, your school counselor or call

CRISIS HOTLINE
228-1505

Suicide prevention is everyone's responsibility.

FIGURE 8.1. "Crisis card" issued to students in the high school after the suicide of S.

A number of teachers were identified as particularly upset about the two suicides, as they had taught both students. I scheduled a meeting after school with teachers to discuss coping, but no one attended. It is interesting to note that the next morning one of the teachers commented on how hard it was to come to school and noted that he had experienced a suicide in his family. I stated that I understood. He questioned my ability to understand; I replied that I, too, was a survivor of suicide, and then we had a very meaningful and supportive discussion. I told him that I had been very upset on the way to school, but had used a lot of positive self-talk to convince myself that I not only could cope but could help others cope as well!

An assistant principal brought me a draft of the student newspaper, which featured an article on suicide. I had two major concerns about the article: First, it did not focus enough on prevention, and second, it did not stress the necessity to break a confidence and get help for a suicidal friend. The article interviewed four students and asked them that very question; two of the four students responded, "No, you should not tell an adult about the suicidal thoughts and plans of your friend." I was horrified. I reworked the article, emphasizing prevention, and instructed the journalism teacher to take those two student responses out. The question about telling adults was answered for students in the affirmative and the answers of two other students who gave the right answer were substituted. I offered to talk with the two students who would now not have their pictures in the paper. They were polite but upset, and maintained that they would still not tell an adult. One student actually came around slightly, but then supported the other student's viewpoint. I stated that I was sorry that I couldn't convince them, but that I felt that friend intervention and getting the assistance of an adult were vitally important in preventing youth suicide. I reminded them of the recent court ruling that schools can exercise editorial control over student newspapers.

A number of other students were identified as suicidal, and some low-lethality attempts occurred after S's death. Many parents called and asked what the school was doing and how they could help their children. Most calls were positive, but a few were critical of the school: The academic climate at the school was criticized, and some teachers were reported as uncaring. One call reported a rumor of a suicide pact involving the two deceased students and others. I recommended to the principal and the counseling staff that we have a parent meeting. I stated that I thought that a proactive stance was advisable, rather than waiting for the parents and community to demand an accounting of what the school was doing. Everyone agreed, although one counselor mentioned bringing in some outside experts. I disagreed with that suggestion and recommended that we do it, as I felt that we were on top of the situation. We needed to present our district procedures and the steps that we had taken at the school. I was very concerned about what message we would be giving the parents by bringing in outside experts.

A letter was mailed to all parents, which acknowledged the two suicides and invited parents to attend a presentation entitled "Suicide Prevention Is Everyone's Responsibility." Parents were encouraged to bring their children.

I prepared extensively for the parent meeting. The principal, the counseling team leader, and I had several planning meetings. The strategy that we decided on emphasized the following:

1. The school cared and had been very responsive to this societal problem. The district's suicide intervention program was outlined.

2. My credentials and work in this area were emphasized.

3. Postvention was described as a team effort.

4. The focus was on coping for the school community and preventing further suicides, not on specifics about method and causation in these two suicides.

5. The goal was to provide all who attended the meeting with the facts about suicide and how they could prevent it. Numerous handouts were provided.

6. Parents who were critical of our efforts were asked to become active in advising us.

The following outline specifies the topics that were covered and by whom. It was very important that the principal begin and end the meeting. The counseling staff initially did not want to take an active role in the presentation. They changed their minds, however, and this helped promote a team response from administrators, counselors, and psychologists.

    I. Welcome, we care—Principal

   II. Overview of suicide and how to prevent it—Director of psychological services (myself)

  III. Summary of district suicide intervention program—Director of psychological services

  IV. Postvention at the high school—Counselor team leader

   V. Warning signs, myths, and situational nature of suicide—School psychologist

  VI. Communication between parents and teenagers—Director of psychological services

 VII. Community resources—School psychologist

VIII. Questions—All

We were uncertain how many parents and teenagers might attend such a meeting. The letter announcing the meeting was mailed to all 2,500 students' parents. One question that I was asked was whether or not the marquee in front of the school should announce the meeting. I thought not, as we had notified all parents, and I did not want every passing motorist to link suicide and the school. There was no media coverage of either suicide. Approximately 350 parents and teenagers attended the meeting, along with the superintendent, several school board members, and the family of G. I had kept the superintendent briefed on postvention steps, and he had kept the school board informed. The superintendent was very interested in postvention efforts. He informed me that a local minister had asked to address the entire student body of the high school. The superintendent had declined the request, but asked that I call and discuss the situation with the minister. It was threatening to me to see the superintendent and school board members in attendance.

I opened my remarks by emphasizing that this was the largest group with which I had ever had the opportunity to talk about suicide prevention, and that this was a tribute to their concern and caring. I outlined that we would be focusing on grief resolution and prevention. Specifics about the two suicides would not be discussed. I also stressed that my comments and recommendations to them were based on years of research and study, and not just on what I knew about these two students and their deaths. I acknowledged that I was a survivor of suicide, and thus had some understanding of their emotions.

The meeting, which lasted about 90 minutes, went very well. I stressed the situational nature of suicide and empowerment. I shared a success story at the close of my remarks. All the presenters did a good job. The parents and teenagers were very attentive. The presentation was filmed by the high school so that it would be available to parents and students who could not attend. There was only one difficult question, and it was the first one. A parent stated, "I understand that both of these students had received psychological help, and they still committed suicide. How do you explain that?" I replied that it would be inappropriate for me to discuss specific things about these two young people; it would be a violation of their respective families' privacy. I reminded the parent that what I was recommending to the group was based on years of study. I emphasized very strongly that professional assistance could mean the difference between life and death for a suicidal youth. The rest of the questions were easy to answer, and several parents and teenagers said very positive things about the postvention efforts at the school.

A school counselor outlined a project in which students were interested. The project would create a helpline at the high school that students could call. Parents and students who were interested in supporting this project were encouraged to sign up. The principal thanked everyone for attending and adjourned the meeting. We received very prompt and positive feedback from the superintendent and G's family. G's father mentioned that he thought about making some comments, but was afraid that his comments might have gotten us off the positive emphasis on looking forward and preventing further suicides.

These two suicides were very difficult for the school community. The impact on the student body was significant. One counselor commented, "Every day we identify two or three more suicidal students." The school and especially the counseling staff stayed very focused on postvention activities, which resulted in the prevention of further suicides. Numerous students were referred for services in the community, and a few were even hospitalized. Gradually, however, things returned to normal, and suicidal students are now identified once or twice a week rather than several a day.

POSTVENTION PROCEDURES

The school becomes a focal point for a tremendous amount of attention after a student's suicide. Postvention procedures should be written and clearly understood by all concerned. Johnson and Maile (1987) stress the school's resources and its opportunity to promote healing through postvention. They comment, "Without exception, the most effective and consistent response comes from schools that are prepared. Advance training and preparation for dealing with grief and fear increases the probability that such healing will occur" (1987, p. 210). Schools have humanistic personnel who have the trust of their students and the time necessary to process events and help students cope with their emotions. Lamb and Dunne-Maxim (1987) emphasize that early intervention through planned interventions with survivors can facilitate grief resolution. The school community, like the surviving family, often responds with immense grief, guilt, anger, and distortion of the truth. The main concern of the school administration is that another student will imitate the suicide. Hill (1984) notes that the schools provide a viable location for postvention work, and stresses the responsibility that school faculty members often feel to do something after a suicide to help students cope. Hill states,

A student had committed suicide. The very fact that it was a student brought focus on the school. What might the school have done (or failed to do) to have averted this death? Now that there had been a death, the school was under implicit, and sometimes explicit, pressure to do something. Such pressure came from within as well as outside the school system. (1984, p. 408)

School administrators have good intentions, but usually have had no training in suicide prevention, let alone postvention. The most frequent strategy is to pretend that the suicide did not happen and to hope that no other suicides occur. Crabb (1982) notes that administrators want to get back to normal and that counselors in particular may have to be advocates for providing opportunities at school for students to express their emotions. Crabb stresses that students need open and honest communication that confronts the crisis, not false assurances that everything will be alright. These feelings can be expressed through artwork, music, and writing, in addition to small classroom discussions.

Lamb and Dunne-Maxim (1987) state that schools need to be kept open and seen as functioning as much as possible. Normal procedures that the school follows in the event of a death should be followed, care should be taken not to glorify or romanticize the death by suicide in any way. Dunne-Maxim (1987) provides an example of a principal who refused to fly the school flag at half-mast after a student committed suicide. The decision upset many grieving students, as this was a routine observation of a death in the school community. Since this was the normal procedure at the school, I would have flown the flag at halfmast.

The suicide prevention guide published by the Wisconsin Department of Instruction (1986) makes a number of postvention recommendations:

- Don't dismiss school or encourage funeral attendance during school hours.
- Don't dedicate a memorial to the deceased.
- Don't have a large assembly.
- Do give the facts to the students.
- Do emphasize prevention and everyone's role.
- Do provide small-group counseling.
- Do emphasize that no one is to blame for the suicide.
- Do emphasize that help is available and that there are alternatives to suicide.

Several writers have stressed the disruptiveness of the suicide of a student and the profound impact that it can have on the school community. The primary task of postvention is grief resolution. This does not necessarily conflict with the administrative goal of a return to normality. My experience has been that a return to normality can best be accomplished through planned activities that provide opportunities for students and faculty to talk about their feelings and to become involved in meaningful activities to help others. Several key guiding principles should be followed:

1. School should be perceived as continuing.
2. Normal procedures in the aftermath of a death should be followed as much as possible. The death and the fact that it was a suicide should be acknowledged. It is not necessary or advisable to give details of the method used.
3. The faculty members should be provided coping assistance first; they will then be better able to help students cope.
4. Care should be taken not to romanticize or glorify the death.
5. Networking efforts should provide both individual and group counseling to the close friends of the deceased and other students known to have been suicidal before.
6. Small classroom discussion, presentations, and announcements are preferable to a large school assembly.
7. It is appropriate to contact the family, and support from the school will be appreciated.
8. Funeral attendance by faculty and students should be in accordance with the procedure for other deaths; however, it is preferred that the funeral not be held during school hours.
9. Memorials and remembrance should be downplayed, with no school activities, plaques, or the like dedicated. It is suggested that donations be sent to a national organization for the prevention of youth suicide or put in a general scholarship fund.
10. Extreme care should be taken with media contact, and written procedures for dealing with the media are recommended. (See Chapter 9.)
11. Counselors and administrators who are dealing with the crisis should meet frequently and debrief.

Dunne-Maxim (1987) has addressed the question of whether or not such planning and the development of a suicide intervention program create or cause suicidal behavior or suicides. The answer is no, and it is recommended that school systems write policies utilizing the resources of the school and the community in the area of postvention.

FREQUENTLY ASKED QUESTIONS ABOUT POSTVENTION

Q. *Should the suicide be acknowledged?*
A. Yes. There is a consensus that the death should be acknowledged as a suicide. Lamartine (1985) notes that administrators are reluctant to do

so; however, if the suicide is not acknowledged, other students who are suicidal may feel that their own suicidal thoughts and actions should not be revealed.

Q. *Should special activities be planned for the entire school faculty?*
A. Yes. The faculty should be notified as soon as possible, utilizing a calling tree. A faculty meeting should be held as soon as possible. Faculty members will need assistance in coping with their own emotions. Some may feel guilty, because they now realize that there were clues to the suicide (Lamartine, 1985). Some faculty members can even be scapegoated by others and seen as having put too much pressure on the student who committed suicide (Dunne-Maxim, 1987). The faculty meeting can guide teachers toward not only working through their own feelings, but modeling expression of feelings for students. Hill (1984) and Lamb and Dunne-Maxim (1987) emphasize that the faculty is not as open to talking about the suicide as the peer group.

Q. *What are the primary tasks of postvention?*
A. Grief resolution for the school community and prevention of further suicides. Worden (1982) has outlined the tasks of grief resolution as follows: to accept the reality of the loss; to experience the pain of the loss; to adjust to the environment where the deceased is missing; and to reinvest emotions in another relationship.

Grief resolution takes varying amounts of time, and a number of stages are worked through. Kubler-Ross (1969) describes stages of denial, anger, bargaining, depression, and acceptance. She notes that the initial shock or numbness lasts approximately 2–3 days, followed by several weeks of painful longing and preoccupation with memories and mental images of the deceased. She stresses that grief resolution takes from 3 to 12 months. Smith (1985) believes that the mourning process may take as long as 2 years.

Q. *Should opportunities be provided for students to talk about the suicide?*
A. There is a consensus among suicidology experts that students should be told about the suicide and should be allowed to talk about it. There is debate about what format is best.

Q. *Should parents be notified by letter about the suicide?*
A. Yes. This strategy aids in dispelling rumors and facilitates important communication between parents and teenagers on this topic.

Q. *Should a large assembly approach be utilized?*
A. No. Several suicidologists caution against such an approach (Dunne-Maxim, 1987; Eyeman, 1987; Smith, 1985). They recommend a small-group approach. My personal experience has been that a classroom

approach is best. Students will be unlikely to express feelings in a large assembly. There is debate on this particular issue, as Boggs (1987) recommends an assembly approach. Attendance at the assembly is recommended, and the person's name, circumstances, and method of death are all given. This is done to dispel rumors. The feelings of the survivors are focused on, as well as the general thinking of suicidal people and how they feel their death might affect others. A large school assembly, if held, should provide a format for students who are not comfortable speaking up in a large group to ask for assistance. Sources of help should be identified, and students can be given a note card to fill out to ask for help.

Q. *What should be said to the surviving students about the person who committed suicide?*

A. Two suicidologists (Eyeman, 1987; Garfinkel, 1986) recommend stressing the psychopathology of the completer. It is important that survivors know that the adolescent who committed suicide had problems unique to him or her. Eyeman feels that the greater the extent to which the completer is portrayed as maladaptive and different from the norm, the less likely it is that modeling effects will occur. Garfinkel believes that emphasizing the problems of the suicide victim demystifies suicide. This approach makes a lot of sense, especially when the suicide victim was well liked and admired and was viewed by other students as having a lot going for him or her. It is vitally important that great care and tact be utilized in stressing the psychopathology of completers to their survivors. I do not recommend this approach to a large group. It may be best utilized in individual counseling with survivors.

Q. *How much opportunity should be provided to talk about the suicide?*

A. Hill (1984) stresses that the makeup of individual teachers, their closeness to the deceased, and their willingness to talk about the death are all factors. A balance needs to be found between acknowledging the tragedy and meeting the demands of the curriculum. Lennox (1987) notes the need for structure, and recommends that classes be held and that students not be allowed to talk about the suicide endlessly. Teachers who are not comfortable with leading a classroom discussion may want to let students express their thoughts through writing. Smith (1985) feels that students need to talk about the suicide and memories that they have of the deceased. Students will also be very interested in details of the suicide and in searching for the reasons why the person committed suicide. I have observed these reactions and feel that some discussion aids acceptance and resolution of the death. Discussion that dwells on the details of a death should be avoided. Smith emphasizes that school personnel need to identify and reflect the anger, guilt, sadness, and anxiety feelings that are part of their grief, and to provide continuing support.

Q. *Who is most at risk of copying the suicide?*

A. Two groups are at risk. The first consists of those students who have been suicidal before, regardless of whether or not they were close to the victim. The second group consists of the close friends of the victim. These two groups should be the focus of more intensive assistance from counselors, school psychologists, and mental health professionals. Both small-group and individual counseling should be available to these students.

Q. *Will all students at the school react in the same way?*

A. No. Students need to be given permission for a wide range of emotions. Teachers and students should refrain from getting angry at those students who do not display the most obvious signs of grief, such as crying. Some students may laugh or make sardonic comments that suicide is stupid. Students may also try to distance themselves from what occurred so that they do not have to deal with unresolved issues surrounding prior losses. Hill (1984) describes situations where students became angry at other students believed to be taking advantage of the situation and pretending to be grieving to get out of class; I have also observed this.

Q. *Who is to blame for the death?*

A. This question will be asked frequently and overtly by teenagers. Adults will think about placing blame but may not overtly discuss it. Dunne-Maxim (1987) reports that the school tends to blame the parents and the parents tend to blame the school. Hill (1984) stressed that teenagers think about what they themselves did or didn't do that caused the death, and they also look externally—toward others at school, the victim's family, or forces in society—to place blame. Lamb and Dunne-Maxim (1987), in noting the importance of group processing, comment, "The message must be that everyone is hurting and everyone is angry—we are all survivors in the same boat. While we will probably never know fully why, we must stop blaming each other and stop blaming ourselves" (p. 259). Lamb and Dunne-Maxim state that it is helpful to cite Shneidman's (1985) thoughts on causation: "[S]uicide is a multifaceted event and biological, cultural, sociological, interpersonal, intrapsychic, logical, conscious and unconscious, and philosophical elements are present in various degrees in each suicidal event" (p. 252). It seems to be no one's and everyone's fault.

Q. *What about funeral attendance?*

A. Normal procedures concerning funeral attendance should be followed for both faculty and students. The ideal situation would be to recommend that the funeral not take place during school hours, to minimize glorifying the death. I have requested of parents that they schedule the service after school or on a Saturday. I have usually found parents to be very understanding.

Q. *What key point should be stressed to the student body and the school faculty for the future?*

A. Everyone should be reminded of the warning signs of suicide and the importance of getting help at once for a suicidal individual. All concerned should be empowered with the belief that they can make a difference—that they can save a life and prevent a future suicide. Students and faculty should be familiar with school referral procedures and community sources of help.

Q. *Should the school personnel contact the victim's family?*

A. Yes. This is a very sensitive issue and one that school systems may shy away from. Contact needs to be made with the student's parents for many reasons. The school system should initiate the contact. Lamb and Dunne-Maxim (1987) stress that the school can and should express condolences in a formal, face-to-face manner. This meeting allows for a return of personal items that belong to the student and provides the opportunity to discuss the funeral and memorials to the deceased with the family. In addition, I have been aware of several situations in which siblings of the deceased attended our schools and were in need of immediate and long-term assistance; directly approaching the parents facilitated our providing the siblings with this help. School personnel can also help direct the family to assistance available in the community, such as survivor groups. The school needs to recognize the fact that the families of those who commit suicide have historically been ostracized. Dunne-Maxim (1987) notes that survivors are prone to guilt and that their plan and loss is compounded by the stigma that they feel. This stigma has resulted in many families' denying the suicide for months or even years. I have worked with students who found out years later what the real circumstances were concerning the death of a relative. The stigma that our society has attached to the survivors of suicide will not go away easily, but a caring, reaching-out response from the school is a first step.

Q. *Can students assist the family of the victim?*

A. Yes. Lindeman and Greer (1972) stress how valuable the peer group can be in helping the family of the deceased. Hill (1984) points out that our society is reluctant to express emotions after a death, especially after a suicide. Any attempt by the peer group to reach out to parents will be most appreciated. School faculty can model reaching out to the family.

Q. *In what way should the student who committed suicide be memorialized?*

A. The school system should not glorify or sensationalize the death in any way. This can best be accomplished by following normal procedures as much as possible. I have had the opportunity to recommend that funds go to a worthy cause, such as scholarship funds or suicide prevention efforts. Schools have been requested to dedicate yearbooks, dances, and a variety of other school events to the deceased; the answer to such requests should be no. Students may want to do something in the form of a project, and with careful monitoring they may be allowed to do this. Lamb and Dunne-Maxim (1987) comment, "In general, the emphasis should be on moderating institutional responses to avoid overdramatization. Instead, the focus must be on the needs of the living, the survivors" (p. 249). They also recommend against any kind of physical memorial at school.

Q. *What about a presentation to other parents?*

A. The school should be ready and willing to provide a supportive and educational meeting to parents following a suicide of a student. From a public relations standpoint, it would behoove the school to volunteer to hold a meeting for parents, instead of waiting until the community demands it. My experience with such meetings has been positive. Attendance has varied from a few parents to several hundred. The parents who attend get a lot of valuable information from it that might prevent another suicide. A proactive approach is recommended, with school personnel rather than outside experts making the presentations to parents, if at all possible.

Q. *In terms of postvention resources, what is needed? Should an outside consultant be called in?*

A. Not necessarily. It is very important that the school system contact someone familiar with postvention or have someone on staff who has had experience with it. Lamb and Dunne-Maxim (1987) recommend that a consultant be brought in from a mental health center. Most of the articles that have been written about postvention in the schools have been written by outside consultants. The need for an outside consultant depends on the circumstances of the suicide and on the resources and preparation of the school system. The professional experienced in postvention can provide much needed leadership. Pelej and Scholzen (1987) caution against relying on an expert to handle the crisis; they stress that the school crisis team should handle it. The California State Department of Education (1987) recommends an outside expert. I personally believe that efforts should be made to train and utilize school personnel.

SUICIDE AT SCHOOL

Several school districts have dealt with the impact of having a student commit suicide on school grounds and in front of other students. Having the suicide occur at school intensifies the situation for all concerned. Gumbleton and Eichinger (1987) and Jackson (1988) have discussed dealing with such an incident. Gumbleton and Eichinger (1987), who are school psychologists, describe an incident in Los Angeles in which an 18-year-old Salvadoran immigrant shot himself in front of 35 students in an English-as-a-second-language class. Jackson, also a school psychologist, discusses the reaction of students in a math class in Katy, Texas (near Houston) who witnessed a 15-year-old boy shooting himself to death.

Gumbleton and Eichinger (1987) had to overcome language barriers, but provided the class with extensive opportunities to discuss the incident during subsequent school days. The students had a pronounced shock reaction and had much difficulty dealing with the visual image of what had happened. Gumbleton and Eichinger describe how important it was to work with the group of students at school over a several-day period to build trust and to help them process the incident. The students progressed to assimilating the incident and voted to rearrange the chairs in the classroom; they were eventually able to get on with their school work.

Jackson (1988) discusses the overwhelming media response to the incident in Katy: The local news media sent helicopters to the school. Students were angry, shocked, and confused. Jackson had previously worked on suicide intervention and the development of district procedures. This preparation resulted in a crisis team approach and much support being immediately provided to students and faculty. The students who witnessed the shooting were immediately and permanently moved to another classroom, and were kept together and worked with for the remainder of the school day. Follow-up in the class period where the shooting happened was provided for several weeks. The students later participated in a reality-oriented physical exercise program emphasizing teamwork. A meeting for parents was also held at the school. Jackson notes that the girls who had witnessed the incident showed more emotion than the boys. Jackson stressed how valuable the prior planning and training in crisis intervention were in the school's being able to handle an incident of this magnitude.

Jackson (1988) and Gumbleton and Eichinger (1987) do not specify exactly what strategies they employed to help students overcome and manage the violent visual images. A technique that I have used with survivors is to have them replace the violent image of the deceased with a pleasant memory. I also recommend limiting the amount of time that they spend visualizing the suicide. A suicide at school will greatly heighten the need for an organized, multifaceted postvention response from the crisis team.

CHILDREN AS SURVIVORS AT SCHOOLS

Schools need to be prepared to reach out and assist children who are survivors of a suicide. Dunne-Maxim, Dunne, and Hauser (1987) have addressed the question of how many such children there are in the United States. They point out that when one includes the suicides of parents, aunts, uncles, grandparents, siblings, and close friends, the number is quite large. Small and Small (1984) have estimated the figure at 350,000–600,000 child survivors. Dunne-Maxim et al. (1987) feel that this figure is an underestimate.

School children who survive a suicide are going to need postvention assistance. I have found child survivors to be most appreciative of support. Dunne-Maxim et al. (1987) point out that these children often suffer from posttraumatic stress syndrome because of the unexpected, violent nature of suicide. Characteristics that these children may exhibit are as follows: cognitive–perceptual difficulties and distortion of the suicide; foreshortened and pessimistic sense of their future; problems in their own developmental accomplishments and feelings of shame about the suicide; and repetitive dreams of the suicide.

Children need to be told openly and honestly about the suicide. I vividly remember telling my son about the suicide of his grandfather. I waited until he was 8, because I was not sure that he would understand earlier. I also had begun being more open in my disclosure with others, and I did not want him to hear about it from anyone else. I will never forget his first comment: "You lied to me, because you told me that he had a heart attack!" I clarified that my father had suffered a heart attack before his suicide. I had led my son to believe that his grandfather died of a heart attack, but I had planned to give him specifics when he was old enough to understand. My son seemed to grasp the logic behind this and asked a number of questions about his grandfather's mental health and the circumstances. As a parent, I feel relief that he now knows the truth, and when he occasionally asks a question or two about suicide I answer them.

Children need to know the facts, and the sooner the better. Child survivors often become very interested in learning about suicide. I believe that we need to assist them in their search for knowledge.

Parents and family members may attempt to shield child survivors from some aspects of the funeral rituals, and may be so caught up in their own needs that they do not attend to the children. Surviving children need guidance on what to expect when they return to school, especially how to respond to questions; they need to be told that they have nothing to feel ashamed about. They also need follow-up support. I am presently meeting weekly with two adolescent survivors. I have met with them individually up to this point, but we are about to begin meeting as a small group. The two students are very excited about the three of us meeting together. They have much in common with regard to school and the grieving process.

Dunne-Maxim et al. (1987) note that a surviving child often actually increases his or her efforts at school in an attempt to become a model child. Issues that I have been aware of have been somewhat different: They have centered around concentration difficulty, loss of motivation in school, preferring to be with friends instead of family, feeling overprotected, and feeling pressured to accomplish more than before the suicide. One student commented, "It's like walking on eggshells at home. I don't know whether to bring up my brother who committed suicide or not. I spend a lot of time in my room."

Schools need to be compassionate to survivors with regard to academic performance. One high school student who survived his sibling's suicide had difficulty concentrating and failed science each grading period after the suicide. I encouraged the teacher to give the student a grade based on the grading periods before the suicide. This enabled the teacher in good conscience to pass the student. Teachers sometimes do not understand how traumatic it is to survive a suicide and may expect too much too quickly with regard to academic performance.

Iris Bolton, who is herself a survivor of a suicide, has written much on the topic. She has compiled a list of suggestions from the survivors with whom she has worked. These suggestions from Bolton (1987), which are summarized below, have relevance for school personnel.

1. You can survive, although you will never be the same. All feelings are normal and do not mean that you are crazy. You are in mourning.
2. Suicidal thoughts are common, and you don't have to act on them.
3. Take one day at a time and find a good listener. Crying is okay.
4. The choice to commit suicide was theirs, not yours. It is okay to be angry at them.
5. Put off major decisions and expect some setbacks.
6. Get professional help.
7. Get all those questions and feelings out.

Schools can provide much assistance to child survivors. I have found families and the surviving children themselves to be very appreciative.

SCHOOL HELPLINES OR HOTLINES

A logical response of students at school who want to do something about youth suicide is to create a hotline or helpline. Several such helplines exist. The *Report of the School Suicide Programs Questionnaire* (Smith et al., 1987) indicated that approximately one-fourth of the respondents reported some type of peer counseling program.

Lipton and Leader (1985) have discussed 5 years of operation of a hotline in California called the Teen Line. They point out that this is a logical way to reach troubled teens, due to their familiarity with telephones. The telephone is immediate and available, and is an equalizer of social, economic, and societal differences. The Teen Line model developed by Lipton and Leader emphasizes active listening in a caring, empathetic, and nonjudgmental manner. Teenagers who want to answer calls are screened and participate in 18 hours of training. They are then assigned to one 4-hour shift per week for a minimum of 6 months. Ongoing supervision is provided to the teens who answer the Teen Line. Lipton and Leader (1985) comment,

> The Teen Line model in no way substitutes for or competes with a professional evaluation and intervention. It does offer immediate contact with a caring and concerned other, and the potential for issue clarification and resolution and referral. For the adolescent in pain, that can be life saving. (p. 222)

I have been involved with several helpline projects, most recently at the high school where two suicides occurred (see "Case Study 2," this chapter). Students tend to think in terms of a major project that will really make an impact. One girl asked in a planning meeting, "How many suicides did the last helpline prevent?" I had to answer, "None that I know of, but no suicides occurred during that week." She then asked, "How many calls did the helpline get?" I said, "Very few." I went on to emphasize, however, that the students who received the training got a lot out of it. I think that one of the major objectives of a helpline should be to provide valuable training to the volunteers. A helpline project also needs to be planned carefully, and students need to realize that it is an ambitious project.

Some people would question whether a high school should do such a project at all. One teacher did not support the most recent helpline project and would not recommend students for it, because she felt that students who answered the phone would be in a most difficult position. I feel that teenagers are in that position every day without training or adult supervision. Another question is whether the students or the school could be sued. I know of no lawsuits that have been filed for this reason. Still another question is that of how much training students should receive to be able to answer the phones. Crisis hotline volunteers receive as much as 40 hours of training; that is a lot of training to expect a high school student to go through before he or she can answer a school helpline.

The following steps were taken to plan the most recent high school helpline:

1. A planning team of students set the helpline as a goal. A counselor and teacher assisted.
2. Several meetings presented the team with an overview of youth suicide.
3. Students were recruited to work on the project.
4. The student body was surveyed to see whether the helpline would be used; 40% said yes.
5. Students who wanted to be trained to work on the helpline had to get parental permission and a recommendation from a teacher.
6. Parent volunteers were recruited.
7. School personnel volunteers to supervise the helpline were recruited.
8. An 8-hour training session was held on a Saturday.
9. Helpline objectives were developed.
10. The helpline was made available during the first week of May 1988, which was National Suicide Prevention Week.
11. Administrative support was received from the principal and the superintendent.
12. Completion of the training was a requirement to work on the helpline.
13. Procedures were written to clarify the responsibilities of student volunteers, parent volunteers, and supervising district employees.
14. A publicity committee was formed to promote awareness of the helpline.

The training that the students and parents received emphasized the following:

• Warning signs of suicide
• How to respond to a suicidal friend
• The necessity of adult assistance
• The situational nature of suicide
• Problem solving
• Recognizing and managing stress
• Being a good listener

- Showing empathy and reflecting feelings
- An overview of the citywide hotline and types of calls received
- Telephone intervention skills and etiquette
- Anonymity, objectivity, and the need not to promise to become the caller's friend
- Handling crank calls
- Keeping a record of all calls and notifying the supervisor of all calls at the end of the shift

The training provided numerous role-play opportunities in small groups so that the students could try out these skills. Some students had difficulty going slowly and reflecting feelings; they wanted to move too quickly into advice giving. For example, one student was given the following scenario: "Bill's girlfriend broke up with him, and he has called the helpline." Her first response was to ask, "Why do you think that she broke up with you?" I suggested that she make a feeling statement, such as "That must be difficult for you," or "You are hurt by this." A number of students had problems such as this one; the parents, however, were very supportive and grasped the importance of recognizing feelings. At the end of the day, everyone had improved in this area immensely. One of the parents who had been trained commented, "This information, and especially responding to feelings, is going to help me in my life!"

Everyone who participated in the training received a certificate. The students were so enthusiastic that when it came time to sign up for a shift assignment, there was a stampede. Before we allowed them to sign up, all procedures were reviewed. I emphasized that by signing up, the students were making a commitment to follow the procedures. Each student was assigned to one 3-hour shift during the week. Each shift had one 9th-grader, one 10th-grader, one 11th-grader or 12th-grader, one parent, and one school employee. School employees were primarily counselors or psychologists. Students were given two additional handouts entitled "Hints for Handling Calls" and "Student Volunteer Procedures."

The 1-week helpline project went very smoothly. All students, parents, and faculty completed their shift assignments. There were only six real calls during the week; none of the calls were suicidal in nature. They were, however, about real adolescent problems—school work, drugs, friends, family, and pregnancy. Not every student got to answer a call. The morale of the students was high, and we adults kept reminding them of the project objectives and noting that they should feel good about their commitment to help others. We also reminded them that they had said that if they got one real call, the project was a success.

A follow-up meeting was held with all students who participated in the project. Everyone involved was asked to fill out a survey asking his or her opinion about the project and what should be done in the future. The following are results of the survey:

1. Ninety-one percent viewed the project as a success.
2. One hundred percent would work again on a similar project.
3. Ninety-seven percent felt adequately supervised.
4. Sixty-four percent felt adequately trained to answer the phones.

One future option that is being considered is to make the project a district-wide one and encourage students from the other three high schools and seven junior high schools to use the helpline. Important questions that still remain are how to publicize the helpline, how long to keep it in operation, and how to supervise it. I view the project as a success. The students involved learned a great deal, and they were able to participate in a project that they initiated and to schedule and complete it before the end of school.

CONTAGION

Increasing attention has been devoted in recent years to the concept of contagion and to how the suicide of one young person affects others. Teen suicide clusters have also been identified (see Table 8.1), and these clusters have received much media attention.

School administrators are very concerned about the contagion aspects of suicide. This is the single reason why most school systems do not have postvention policies. Most administrators believe that the safest course is to do nothing at all in the aftermath of the suicide of a student, and they caution against talking openly about the suicide. Durkheim (quoted in Coleman, 1987b, p. 110) commented that "no fact is more readily transmitted by contagion than suicide but its radiating influence is very restricted." Coleman (1987b) points out that the work of Durkheim emphasized that imitation did not affect the suicide rate; as a result, contagion has not received the careful study that is needed. Ross (1985a) stresses the common linking of contagion factors and youth suicide. She notes that psychologists as early as 1845 pointed out the imitation factor in suicide and the fact that children are more suggestible than adults. Ross has reviewed studies on contagion and found no conclusive evidence substantiating the existence of contagion. She comments, "Indeed, it is my feeling that the 'rule of silence' should be relegated to the list of dangerous myths about suicide, because, more than having 'no point,' it even deters any discussion which could be ameliorative" (1985a, p. 154).

TABLE 8.1. Teen Suicide Clusters

Year	Location
1979	Gardner, Maine
	Loveland, Colorado
1980–1981	Fairfax County, Virginia
1982	Suburban Milwaukee, Wisconsin
	Cheyenne, Wyoming
1983	Groveport, Ohio
	Plano, Texas
	Quakertown, Pennsylvania
1984	Santa Barbara, California
	Westchester, Putnam, and Rockland Counties, New York
	Leominster, Massachusetts
	Clear Lake, Texas
	Houston, Texas
1985	Richardson, Texas
	Helena, Montana
	Brainerd, Crosby, and LaCrosse, Minnesota
	Jefferson County, Colorado
	Chicago, Illinois (northwest side)
	Wind River, Wyoming
1986	Omaha, Nebraska
	Spencer, Massachusetts
	North Sioux City, South Dakota
	Mankato, Minnesota
	Clearfield, Utah
1987	Broken Arrow, Oklahoma
	Bethel, Alaska
	Newton, Massachusetts
	Kansas City, Missouri
	Bergenfield, New Jersey, and nationwide
	Chicago area, Illinois
	Indiana (statewide)

Note. Adapted from *Suicide Clusters* (pp. 115–120) by L. Coleman, 1987, Boston: Faber & Faber. Copyright 1987 by L. Coleman. Adapted by permission.

It appears that many people have been so concerned about contagion that they have refused to comment on or acknowledge suicide. Klagsbrun (1976) stresses that young people will not commit suicide because they hear about it, and cautions that overprotecting young people from the topic denies them the help that they need. Boggs (1987) stresses the necessity of talking about the suicide openly. This discussion takes away the mystique that cloaks suicide and makes it less likely that another young person will commit suicide. Smith (1985) recommends an open, meaningful discussion in direct language, with the goal of stabilizing the situation. Boggs notes the survivors' need for an open discussion to gain support, and cautions that a nonsupportive, closed atmosphere in the school may result in students' keeping their suicidal thoughts to themselves and being more likely to follow through on an attempt.

Several writers have commented on the need to provide resources and specific guidance to teenagers so that they can help themselves and others who are suicidal. There does appear to be an imitative or contagion effect in teen suicide, and schools need to recognize this but not to be handicapped by it. The postvention recommendations made in the bulk of this chapter should all be followed in a contagion situation. The school should do more, not less, in a contagion situation. The suicide of a student cannot and should not be covered up, and young people are going to talk about it. The question is whether these discussions will take place with or without the guidance of trained adults. It is important that the discussions be guided to avoid romanticizing and mysticizing the suicide and to avoid dwelling on details of the method employed. Ross in commenting on the existence of imitation factors, states that "the danger of copy-catting does not exist in all teens. Average, happy people are not going to kill themselves" (quoted in Landers, 1987b, p. 16). Ross recommends that postvention efforts concentrate on vulnerable teens who have a history of problems.

The media coverage intensifies when there has been a cluster of suicides. Dunne-Maxim (1987) and Ryerson (1987) have both commented on the intense media attention that Bergenfield, New Jersey, received in spring 1987 following the suicide of four teenagers by carbon monoxide poisoning. The media coverage was overwhelming, with reporters on the scene from as far away as Moscow. Each reporter wanted a story, and the school system was portrayed as at fault to some extent, despite the fact that all four students had dropped out of school. The intensity of the media coverage following a cluster of suicides makes it imperative that media guidelines be in place and be followed by all concerned (see Chapter 9).

How many teenage suicide clusters are there? How many teenage suicides are imitative of the suicide of a friend, an acquaintance, a family member, or even a faculty member? These are logical questions, but there is no way to answer them fully at present. What are the factors that make a teenage suicide cluster more likely to occur? Smith (1985) has addressed this question and identified the following factors that were present in communities where clusters occurred:

- A lack of integration and belonging.
- Patterns of drug and alcohol abuse in children and adults.
- An emphasis on material possessions.
- A lack of supportive relationships.

- A lack of community awareness of suicide as a problem.
- No 24-hour crisis hotlines.
- Rapid, uncontrolled growth in the community.
- A massive school system with large schools.
- A lack of a network effort by community agencies.

Biblarz (1988) stresses that an emotionally charged environment, in which vulnerable teenagers feel that a person who committed suicide has achieved a desired goal, may well contribute to contagion. Barrett (1985b) cites an emphasis on material possessions, uncontrolled growth, and an obsession with competition as community factors.

Comstock (1985) has summarized the reaction of one community (Clear Lake, Texas) that experienced a suicide cluster. The community reacted with initial disbelief and questioned what was wrong with itself. A fearfulness developed that resulted in questioning whether or not the town would survive. This was followed by feelings of outrage and a desire to place the blame on economic conditions, teenage drug usage, or the school system. The media attention that the town received was also resented by the residents. Reporters were everywhere; although they behaved responsibly, their presence contributed to the climate of anxiety and fear. In all the panic and confusion, many professionals in the community who volunteered to assist felt disregarded. Comstock (1985) summarizes the situation thus:

> The suggestion that there was something toxic in the social fabric of the Clear Lake area was evident and problematic. The suggestion that when school students kill themselves the schools must be responsible was equally problematic. The wide press coverage was a problem in itself; and the abundance of volunteers eager to help but not organized to do anything was a fourth problem. (p. 6)

Comstock also notes that the fact that little is known about youth suicide clusters resulted in fear, anxiety, and many bizarre rumors being spread in the community.

Coleman (1987b) has reported on this same community's reaction and the large group meeting that was held to talk with over 500 parents. Some of the parents blamed the problem on the academic pressures imposed by the school system. I have seen television coverage of other public meetings that were held in the midst of teen suicide clusters; a number of those meetings appeared to be very emotional, and much criticism was likewise directed at the school system. The parent meetings that my colleagues and I have conducted have not resulted in blaming the school system. I think the preparation and leadership role that our school district has taken on this societal problem has been recognized by the community, and as a result the school system has not been blamed.

Coleman (1987b) makes several recommendations about what to do following one or more suicides. He suggests that the school be alert to the possibility of a cluster and pay attention to specific details of the death(s), as well as characteristics and groupings of the teenager(s). Coleman cautions against holding a large assembly and suggests downplaying media coverage. A crisis management team should be created involving school and community officials. (I would hope that such a team would already be in place.) Coleman also recommends making both individual and group counseling at school available and reaching out to assist the surviving families. In addition, it is important to publicize the crisis hotline number; if such a hotline does not exist, it should be created. Creating a hotline would be a productive way to involve the concerned mental health professionals in the community.

Comstock (1985) has based a number of recommendations on the experience of the Clear Lake cluster. Comstock emphasizes that the most important lessons of Clear Lake are that planning in advance of a crisis is necessary and that youth suicide clusters are more than just school business. A multiple-agency, community-wide response is needed. The interventions from outside the community should be held to a minimum, and every community needs a skilled public relations person who can facilitate helpful reporting and protect the rights and public image of the community.

9

Dealing with the Media

The schools need to be prepared to deal with media coverage of teen suicide. As described in Chapter 3, I have had the experience of being interviewed about teen suicide. Large school systems have a public information or public relations representative. I have found our own public relations director to be very helpful, and I have learned a great deal from him. He has become very interested in and knowledgeable about teen suicide. One of the points he emphasizes is the importance of cooperating with the media. This is a very important point, and certainly each school would like to be portrayed by the media as concerned, responsive, and working on the problem of teen suicide. A point that needs to be emphasized to administrators is that there is an immediate linking of a suicide victim and the school that he or she attended. A newspaper headline often identifies the school that the deceased attended. The school is also the first place the media will go for more information; the media do not usually approach the family directly for details. There is no substitute for preparation in any crisis situation, and it is vitally important to be prepared to deal with the media.

There is considerable variation in the emphasis the media will place on a suicide. Teen suicide in general is a major news story only a few times a year. However, it is almost always a major news story when a cluster or series of suicides occurs in the same geographical area, or when two teenagers make a pact and commit suicide together. One teenage suicide in a large city will not receive television, radio, or newspaper coverage as a general rule; by contrast, a teenage suicide in a small community will certainly receive local media attention. Ryerson (1987) stresses the importance of establishing a positive relationship between the media and the school system prior to a crisis. The AAS also recommends a proactive approach and one based upon trust. The interviewee should avoid being defensive and should try to be helpful to the reporter.

This chapter makes a number of recommendations for dealing with the media. The general philosophy that is recommended emphasizes preparation, written procedures, and strategies for positively influencing the media coverage. The school system should also strive to be viewed as recognizing the part that schools play in working on the societal problem of youth suicide. The school system and the media do have some inherent differences, according to Dunne-Maxim (1987): The media want a story, and the school system feels that the less publicity the better.

GUIDELINES FOR DEALING WITH THE MEDIA

1. A written policy should outline procedures to be followed. The policy should specify who will speak with the media representatives.

2. The spokesperson should have a thorough understanding of the dynamics of youth suicide and should be selected because of personal characteristics that enable him or her to represent the school system well.

3. The spokesperson should try to ascertain in advance the types of questions that the media will ask. If it is not possible to ascertain questions in advance, then emphasis should be placed on anticipation of questions. Television interviews will be brief, and it is important to be succinct and to the point.

4. The suicide of the student should be honestly acknowledged, with brief identifying information such as age, grade, and the like provided. The method of suicide should be downplayed.

5. Emphasis should be placed on the steps that the school is taking to assist other students to cope with the suicide. Networking efforts, counseling services, and resources both at school and in the community should be outlined.

6. The problem of youth suicide should be acknowledged, and the prevention efforts that the school system has previously made in this area should be outlined, with documentation provided.

7. The spokesperson should ask the media representative to emphasize the warning signs of suicide and the sources of assistance available at school and in the community. The media should be encouraged to downplay the suicide; to avoid making suicide front-page news; and to avoid simplistic, romantic, or mystic references to the cause of the suicide. An example of the type of headline that should be avoided is this one from the *Springfield* (Missouri) *News-Leader*: "Bright, Popular Ozark Student Falls to Dark, Lonely Thoughts" (1985). The actions of the deceased should not be portrayed as heroic in any way.

8. The media representatives should be escorted around the school building, and access to students should be limited.

9. The spokesperson should emphasize that students are being encouraged to continue with normal school activities as much as possible.

DISCUSSION

Some schools have refused to give interviews on the subject of teen suicide, or have had someone read a prepared statement. Vidal (1986), in fact, recommends reading a prepared statement and giving no personal information about the student. The media, however, may interpret such an approach as uncooperative and indicative of attempting to hide a lack of preparation for the problem of youth suicide. The guidelines offered above should result in more positive information being given to the public about warning signs and sources of help, as well as in better public relations for the school. The designation of a media spokesperson for the school district or individual school enables the spokesperson to improve his or her ability to work with the media and to form a relationship with media representatives. Emphasis should be placed on the very valuable role that the media can play. The school system should approach the media contact in a positive and prepared way, and not as something or someone to be avoided or dreaded. The media contact is an opportunity to promote ways in which youth suicide can be prevented.

Ring (1985) recommends building a cooperative relationship with the media, in the understanding that they have a job to do. The family of the suicide victim should be contacted by the school spokesperson to emphasize that confidentiality has been maintained. This contact, according to Ring, can avoid misunderstandings between the family and the school and can be very beneficial to the family. The family may even choose to make a statement via the school spokesperson. Ring (1985) also discusses the importance of not trying to "stonewall" the media and comments in part, "Attempting to stop reporters from doing their job is how [stonewalling is] perceived. Express the sorrow of the faculty and student body, [and] explain what is being done in the school to deal with the reaction" (p. 40).

The AAS is working on responsible guidelines for media reporting of suicide, as the result of media requests for such guidelines. Preliminary guidelines have been developed by the AAS Public Information Committee and appear in Table 9.1. These guidelines are intended to reduce the possible contagion effects of a suicide. They also deal primarily with a completed suicide and not a suicide attempt; the number of suicide attempts makes it unlikely that an attempt will attract media attention. If the media does inquire about suicide attempts, then the same general

TABLE 9.1. AAS Proposed Media Guidelines

1. Avoid details of the method.
2. Do not report the suicide as unexplainable or the result of simplistic or romantic causes.
3. Avoid making the story front-page news and avoid the word "suicide" in the headline.
4. Do not print a photograph of the deceased.
5. Refrain from coverage that excites or sensationalizes.
6. Do not imply approval of suicide.
7. Simple language should be used and statistics should be reviewed so accurate information is conveyed. Be prepared to cite sources.
8. Be cautious about putting the interviewer in contact with a survivor or an attempter. Get approval from them prior to giving the reporter a name.
9. Avoid discussing the specifics of the situation and safeguard confidential information about your client or student.
10. Include if possible positive outcomes of suicidal crises.
11. Include information on the warning signs, sources of help, and what to do if you detect someone as suicidal.

Note. From "Preliminary Guidelines for Media Developed" by the American Association of Suicidology Public Information Committee, 1987, *Newslink, 13*(2), p. 10. Copyright 1987 by the American Association of Suicidology. Reprinted by permission.

approach should be utilized. One television reporter asked me how many suicide attempts our large school district had each year. Before I could answer, he stated the figure of 25. I just nodded, but thought to myself that the actual figure was probably many times that. I saw no need to alarm the general public and thereby increase the media coverage. Media representatives are generally cooperative and responsible, and I feel that we can have a positive influence on their coverage of youth suicide. I have found them to be very interested in the prevention efforts that our schools have made. They have even gone so far as to take photographs of written procedures and no-suicide contracts. I would not want to be in the position of having to respond to the media coverage of a suicide without being able to produce evidence that the school system has worked on the problem of youth suicide.

The less publicity about circumstances, causation, method, and details of the teenager's life, the better. I wish that teenagers who have sought help and found alternatives to suicide for dealing with the problems of life could receive as much publicity as the teenagers who commit suicide, or that teenagers who intervene and prevent a friend from committing suicide would receive front-page news coverage complete with picture. Phillips (1988) has described convincing a reporter who came out to cover a recent suicide to come back in 6 weeks to do an article on prevention.

10

Curriculum

"Dr. Poland, I agree with everything that you have said about training my school personnel to detect and assist suicidal students, but I don't want to go into the classroom with this topic. Our students in our little old town are pretty silly, and I don't know what they might do!" So said the superintendent of a small school district at the Texas State Superintendents Conference in 1986. As the superintendent's comment indicates, there is considerable debate about whether or not to include suicide prevention as a curriculum topic. Schafly (1985) has very clearly voiced her opposition to suicide prevention as a curriculum topic. Sowers (1988) points out that suicide awareness curriculum programs are in their adolescence and suggests that the programs themselves commit suicide. Sowers expresses concern that suicide awareness programs stand out instead of being well integrated into the curriculum; she also feels that not enough emphasis is placed on coping skills and the overall school climate.

The Samaritans, an international suicide prevention organization, has a different viewpoint. This group has published a book entitled *A Teacher's Manual for the Prevention of Suicide among Adolescents*, edited by Fencik (1986). The foreword to the manual states,

> Because the Samaritans believe that suicide prevention is everybody's business and because we believe that information and education lead to prevention, the following manual was developed with the hope that the information contained therein and shared with students by caring, concerned teachers would reduce the number of adolescent deaths by suicide.

The California State Department of Education agrees: "But it's in the process of learning about suicide that suicidal feelings can be defused"

(1987, p. 4). Suicide prevention education is designed to be implemented in any of several curriculum areas: health, social studies, language arts, physical education, home economics, consumer education, or driver education. It is particularly recommended that classes taken by high school freshmen and sophomores include prevention information. Davis (1985) points out that there is a difference between talking about suicide in the classroom and acting out suicidal thoughts; Davis sees the two as contradictory.

Charlotte Ross was one of the first to advocate suicide as a curriculum topic in the California schools in the 1970s. Ross (1985a) has commented in part,

> The facts of death are as essential to the education of the young—and as intensely sought—as the facts of life. In too many instances, however, there is an additional motivation to learn about suicide. What the increasing rate of youth suicide means to many adolescents is that they know of someone their age who has died by their [sic] own hand. (p. 147)

Ross emphasizes that young people are both attracted and repelled by suicide and will seek out information on their own. I have talked with countless students who hold tightly to dangerous myths about suicidal behavior. The only possible way of getting accurate information about suicide to the many students who need it, and convincing them that suicide can be prevented, is through curriculum presentations.

My own involvement in curriculum development has evolved over a number of years. Few school districts are going to begin a prevention program and include a curriculum component initially. It is a major step simply to get a school district to put something in writing on this topic and to commit itself to a 1- or 2-hour in-service session on detection. The first thought of school administrators is not "Let's address suicide prevention in the curriculum." It would take a state mandate to get most school districts to emphasize prevention in the curriculum. Large school districts that have experienced multiple suicides are doing some work in this area, however.

CURRICULUM DEVELOPMENT: AN EXAMPLE

Chapter 3 relates the case example of the suicide of B. He committed suicide shortly after watching a made-for-television movie on suicide as part of a social studies class. Prior to that time, I had had no idea what, if anything, was being done with regard to suicide as part of the curriculum in my district. After B's death, I saw the need for an in-service training session for health, psychology, and sociology teachers on this topic. I received permission for a 2-hour required session. The in-service training was very much appreciated by the teachers, and they asked for more information. My goal was, from the beginning, to serve as a consultant; it was not my goal to go into the classroom and teach this information myself. My goals for the teachers were to have them do the following:

1. To provide accurate information about the incidence of suicide.
2. To emphasize its situational nature.
3. To dispel the many misperceptions that persist.
4. To teach the warning signs of suicide.
5. To empower students with the knowledge that they can intervene to prevent a suicide and that adults must be notified.
6. To emphasize other alternatives.
7. To familiarize students with assistance available at school and in the community.
8. To promote problem-solving and coping skills.

A follow-up in-service session was planned. This session was approved for advanced academic training credit for teachers. One of the things that I learned was that there are no course objectives or essential elements that deal directly with suicidal behavior or suicide prevention. However, a number of essential elements emphasize such areas as positive mental health, coping with emotions, knowledge of wellness life styles, and problem solving.

An outline of the 6-hour course that I developed, and its objectives, appears below.

Title of Course: Teaching Problem-Solving Skills to Adolescents in the Classroom

Needs Addressed by This Program: Health, sociology, and psychology teachers must help adolescents master essential elements related to their personal well-being, self-concept, goal setting, and ability to understand and overcome social problems such as youth suicide.

Audience for This Program: High school health, sociology, and psychology teachers.

Objectives of the Course: To enhance teachers' ability to teach coping and problem-solving skills and to promote mental health for students.

Descriptions of the Course: Information about goal setting, wellness life styles, and ways in which a student can identify a problem and receive help will be emphasized. How to teach students to cope with stress and emotions and to increase their overall personal well-being will also be included. The warning signs of suicide, and ways in which students can intervene to assist a suicidal friend, will be emphasized.

One of the issues that we dealt with was the question of what suicide-related movies or educational films students should see. Two educational films were recommended and shown. The point was made that educational films were to be preferred over television movies because of their shorter length, which allows for classroom discussion afterwards and minimizes overidentification with the suicidal characters in the films.

Teachers were provided with numerous handouts to use in working with their classes. One of the handouts, which emphasized several key points about suicide education, is presented in Table 10.1.

The psychology department received numerous requests to teach this information in the classroom in the year following this first in-service session. Teachers planned units that varied in length from one to five class periods. Psychologists first responded to requests to teach the unit by offering to consult and help the teachers plan their lessons. The psychologists did agree in some cases to teach the information. I did so, but always with the goal that the teachers would be involved and would feel confident to teach the information on their own the next time. There is one teacher who, each semester, grades papers in the corner of the classroom while a psychologist teaches the information. We continue to try to get this teacher more involved.

MENTAL HEALTH INFORMATION

Should information on mental health be a part of suicide prevention? Yes, I believe very strongly that adolescents need much information about mental health and how to solve problems. First, they should be made aware that they can suffer from emotional problems. Adolescents often discount the fact that they can have emotional problems or negative life experiences (Davis et al., 1988). It is a responsibility of the schools to promote positive mental health, positive self-esteem, future parenting, and citizenship skills, and not just academics. The issue of problem solving, coping, and mental health in general is beyond the scope of this book. Sowers (1987) lists the skills that schools need to teach all students to reduce the likelihood of suicide. The list includes 36 items ranging from human growth and development principles to career selection. Sowers points out that a healthy adolescent needs the following basic skills: self-assessment, communication, decision making, advocacy, and self-management.

TABLE 10.1. Key Points to Remember about Suicide Education

1. Teachers need to be very sensitive regarding *what* they present and *how* they present the facts.
2. Screen all resource materials carefully and have current and factual data.
3. Allow time for discussion of movies or slides. Students need this discussion to process the information.
4. Focus on mental health and problem solving, and not just on suicide prevention, if time permits.
5. Pay attention to the type of questions students ask. If a student exhibits a pattern of interest in suicide, you may want to talk to the student or notify the counselor.
6. Affirm the positive in discussing the topic.
7. Humor is a useful tool in relieving the stress of discussing suicide.
8. Refer students who tell you that they have considered suicide.
9. Warning signs should be emphasized.
10. Guide students who select suicide as a research topic to emphasize prevention and problem solving.
11. Provide students with resources for help: crisis hotline, counseling options, etc.
12. Discuss ideas for helping create a nurturing, safe, and supportive environment at school.
13. Address confidentiality and secrecy directly. When someone's welfare is in jeopardy, we have a responsibility to get help for that person, and this may mean *breaking* a promise not to tell.
14. Scrutinize students' artwork and writing for signs of hopelessness and despair, and refer those students to the counselor.
15. A range of emotions is normal when discussing suicide, and not feeling very much at all is all right as well.
16. Develop a recommended movie list for your school.
17. If one class period is all that you have to devote to suicide prevention, the emphasis should be placed on the warning signs, friend intervention, and the situational nature of suicide.

Cantor (1985) has commented on what schools should focus on: "I would like to see schools set up programs not only on suicide prevention but on how to deal with stress and depression as well, since those are components of suicide and yet adolescents may not address them in the same way that adults do" (p. 87). Barrett (1985b) concludes that curriculum units that are conducted professionally and carefully can have a very positive long-term impact. This point is a good one, and I like to emphasize that knowing the warning signs of suicide and what to do should be looked at as a lifelong skill.

DO CURRICULUM PRESENTATIONS PLANT
THE IDEA OF SUICIDE?

Garfinkel (1986) has criticized programs that focus directly on the topic of suicide prevention and has wondered whether such a direct approach is advisable. The question of whether curriculum presentations plant the idea of suicide in teenagers' minds is a central one in the debate about whether to have such presentations. A number of researchers have answered this question in the negative (Barrett, 1985b; California State Department of Education, 1987; Davis, 1985). Schafly (1985) argues that such presentations do cause more suicides. More research to determine the effects of curriculum presentations has been called for (Berman, 1987b; Ryerson, 1987; Shaffer, 1988).

Ross (1985a), who supports suicide education in the schools, makes the point that adolescents are not innocent and without knowledge about suicide. They are aware of suicide as an option. It does not make sense to me not to deal directly with this topic, given the number of adolescents who think about suicide. A large school district may well have no choice but to include suicide prevention in its curriculum; a small school district that has never experienced a suicide has a choice. I hope that the superintendent of the small school district whose comment opens this chapter will choose to include suicide prevention in the curriculum. If this superintendent and others like him do not do so initially, then I hope that their prevention programs evolve to the point that they will do so in the future. I also hope that superintendents who are making this decision will gather data objectively, and that their judgment will not be impaired by denial and the belief that suicide will not happen in their communities.

THE SITUATIONAL NATURE OF SUICIDE

A key element that must be emphasized in a curriculum presentation is the situational nature of suicide. Students must understand this to see how powerful their interventions can be. Many students have said, "The person who thinks of suicide wants to die and is going to commit suicide sooner or later." These students attach a permanence and eventuality to the decision to commit suicide that simply does not exist. Students need examples of friend interventions and quotes such as these:

> There are times in every man's life when he would like to die temporarily. (Mark Twain)

The man who, in a fit of melancholy kills himself today, would have wished to live had he waited a week. (Voltaire)

The most dramatic illustration that I use involves the Golden Gate Bridge in San Francisco. I talk with students about the beauty of that bridge and the fact that many suicides have taken place there. We discuss suicide in our society and whether bridges should have fences to make it harder to jump or telephones to call crisis hotline centers. I then share with them the following example: "When asked what he thought during his four second fall to the water a survivor recalled thinking, 'I wish I hadn't done this'" (Perlman, 1987, p. 11). Perlman cites statistics showing that of the 515 people who have been stopped from jumping off the Golden Gate Bridge, only 5–6% have later committed suicide. The survivors who were interviewed all stressed that because they were prevented from jumping off the bridge, they developed no other plan to commit suicide.

The situational nature of suicide is also well illustrated in a film entitled *Teens Who Choose Life*, produced by Sunburst Communications (1985). The film consists of three vignettes of teenagers who attempted suicide and survived. The teenagers discuss how fortunate they are to be alive and state that attempting suicide was a poor choice; it almost resulted in a permanent solution to their temporary problem. I have found that showing even one vignette really emphasizes the situational nature of suicide.

An interesting new approach to the concept of situationality uses Shakespeare's *Romeo and Juliet*. Charlotte Ross, the Executive Director of the Youth Suicide National Center, has been working on materials to emphasize alternatives that Romeo and Juliet had to suicide. Working with theatrical experts, Ross has developed other endings to the play, which create an awareness that suicide can be prevented (Harnisch, 1987). More information is available from the Youth Suicide National Center (see Chapter 12 for addresses).

I discussed the question of whether or not Romeo and Juliet should be eliminated, or postponed, from the curriculum given a recent suicide(s) with a former English teacher, Kit Aguren. She feels that the play provides many opportunities to discuss alternatives to suicide, and stressed that the "tragic flaw" of the play is the teenagers' impulsivity and inability to think through the situation. She reported that teenagers are interested in the play but can not identify with the matrimonial customs of the time, in particular with someone meeting and marrying a person after a few days time. I agree with her recommendation that this play be included in the school curriculum (personal communication, 1988).

WHEN SHOULD CURRICULUM PRESENTATIONS BEGIN?

Lennox (1987) asked a number of professionals their opinions as to the age at which curriculum presentations on suicide should begin. Two-thirds favored beginning such units in the fifth, sixth, or seventh grades, with the mean recommendation being grade 6.4.

QUALITIES OF THE TEACHER

What qualities should a teacher have to present information on suicide prevention? Barrett (1985b) stresses the need for the teacher to have worked through his or her thoughts about the right to intervene to save a life. Sensitivity is also emphasized. Lennox (1987) recommends that the teacher have group facilitation skills and a stable personality; concern, sensitivity, and a belief that suicide can be prevented; and availability to follow-up.

Teachers should encourage discussion and let students express their views. Smith (1986) and the Samaritans manual (Fencik, 1986) both emphasize that we cannot force students to change their attitudes. The teacher must give the students time to think about their attitudes and beliefs. Tanney (1988) also stresses that teachers should not be forced to teach this information. Tanney recommends using school personnel as much as possible, instead of bringing in mental health professionals to teach curriculum units.

PARENTAL PERMISSION

What about parental permission for students to participate in curriculum units on suicide? I do not recommend that parental permission be obtained prior to a student's participating in a curriculum program. Parental involvement in advisory groups may be advantageous. The Wisconsin Department of Instruction (1986) cites one program that sends home information to parents about the curriculum presentation but does not ask their permission.

The California State Department of Education (1987) does not require parental permission for its curriculum program. The department comments,

> Some educators and parents may be concerned about the possibility of an outbreak of teenage suicide as a result of talking about it. In truth, the

evidence suggests that not talking about suicide creates barriers for young people who are trying to understand what they are feeling. When you convey a sense of confidence that suicidal feelings are survivable, you are helping students deal with such feelings. (1987, p. 4)

AUDIENCE SIZE

A classroom or homeroom approach is recommended so that there can be interaction and discussion. A large-group, assembly approach is not recommended.

EXAMPLES OF CURRICULUM APPROACHES

Is there one certain approach that a school district should use to develop curriculum materials, or a program that should be adopted in its entirety? Johnson and Maile (1987) stress that few schools adopt a whole program. They emphasize that each school should examine available materials and then decide what fits its particular situation and student body. The *Report of the Suicide Programs Questionnaire* (Smith et al., 1987) concludes that most schools that work on suicide prevention develop their own materials. A number of programs and materials are available, and several are reviewed here to illustrate the most important points to include in the curriculum.

Lifelines

One such program is Lifelines, which was developed by Underwood, Jakubik, and Kalafat in 1985. It consists of a sequential set of preventive educational programs to promote awareness of, and knowledge of ways to prevent and respond to, adolescent suicide. The program provides 6 hours of training to school personnel, who then conduct three class periods on suicide prevention. This curriculum is very straightforward and should be able to address the objectives in the time allotted.

Lifelines provides a consultant who works for a total of approximately 15 hours to train school personnel to carry out the program. The consultant conducts an initial in-service session for administrators and gives them an overview of the program to gain their support and to clarify referral procedures. An overview presentation is also made to interested parents and the entire faculty. The personnel who will be teaching the unit to students are then identified to participate in the 6 hours of training.

Lifelines was developed by school guidance personnel and community education specialists. It is designed to be used with junior and senior high school students and to be implemented in three 45- to 55-minute class periods. The content of the material is educational and problem-centered. Emphasis is placed on teenage stress, friend intervention, and problem solving. Two or three key points are emphasized in each lesson. Active student participation is encouraged, and abstract mental health developmental concepts and jargon are kept to a minimum. Underwood et al. (1985) list two goals for the program: to ensure ready sources of help for suicidal students at school and a rapid response from school personnel; and to provide school staff, students, and parents with knowledge about how to prevent a suicide.

Suicide Prevention Curriculum for Adolescents

A curriculum unit on suicide prevention for adolescents developed by J. Smith (1988b) includes five lesson plans. (The unit can be condensed to three class periods if needed.) Teachers are provided with background information and exercises to stimulate student discussion and to help students master basic lesson concepts. The curriculum unit has five objectives:

1. Students will become aware of their attitudes about suicide.
2. Students will receive correct information about it.
3. Students will learn to detect the warning signs.
4. Students will increase their listening and communication skills.
5. Students will become familiar with sources of help.

Smith stresses the importance of students' participating in the exercises. Smith also emphasizes that suicidal adolescents are crying out for help and that their peers can be taught to respond to save a life.

The first lesson explores attitudes about suicide. Teachers are encouraged to explore their own attitudes before beginning. Smith provides open-ended questions for students to discuss in small groups. Two examples of these questions are as follows:

- Suicide is a problem because . . .
- People who attempt it are . . .

Smith emphasizes that attitudes are to be explored, not taught. The class should close by discussing the feelings stirred up by the lesson.

The second lesson emphasizes the facts about suicide. Each student is provided with a list of 15 true-or-false questions about suicide. Smith stresses that students should understand that this is not a test. After students respond to all items, a discussion of each item is recommended. Sample projects that could be assigned to adolescents are listed, such as reviewing a library book, summarizing a newspaper article on suicide, or gathering information about the local incidence of suicide.

The third lesson focuses on the warning signs. The goal is for every student to be able to identify individuals who are at risk of committing suicide. Smith recommends having students remember a time when they felt miserable. The teacher lists three headings on the blackboard: verbal, behavioral, and situational. Students are asked to talk about their feelings and their behavior. Examples are listed under the appropriate headings on the blackboard. Smith cautions that students should not be forced to participate. A discussion of the known warning signs of suicide follows, with an emphasis on the verbal, behavioral, and situational aspects. Smith recommends showing a film to emphasize the warning signs further. Students should answer questions about warning signs depicted in the films and give reasons why the teenagers were suicidal.

Communication skills are stressed in the fourth lesson. The goal is for students to acquire listening and communication skills that will promote empathetic responses to someone experiencing intense emotions. Exercises are provided to separate thinking and feeling statements. Exercises help students understand that feelings are usually expressed by one word. Students are placed in pairs, and one student reads a sentence while another student identifies his or her feeling. Short role-play activities are also provided to help students identify and reflect feelings and to help them avoid making quick assumptions about the problem, passing judgment, or giving advice. The fifth and final lesson emphasizes friend intervention and knowledge of community resources.

California Suicide Prevention Program

The Suicide Prevention Program for the California Public Schools (California State Department of Education, 1987) contains a lesson guide designed for grades 9 to 12, which includes the following: a curriculum overview; a discussion of special concerns for the teacher; goals and objectives; instructions for lesson preparation, complete lesson plans; student handouts, worksheets, and guides; and supplementary enrichment activities. Overall goals are to increase students' ability to handle their own problems and to respond to troubled friends.

Special concerns are emphasized for the teacher with the comment, "You can't discuss suicide without touching on your own feelings—students' and your own" (California State Department of Education, 1987, p. 3). Discussion of suicide will not burden the students or plant the idea in their heads. The teacher must recognize that this topic needs to be discussed so that students have accurate information, even if someone in the community is not supportive. The following teaching strategies are recommended:

1. Provide structure and ground rules for the class.
2. Recognize cultural differences and protect students' privacy.
3. Give honestly of yourself in the discussions.
4. Be familiar with referral procedures.
5. Stress that everyone is depressed at some time.
6. Be alert and sensitive to students who are upset.
7. Don't try to scare students.
8. Provide some lightness through a positive emphasis and permit some humor.
9. Assist students and be available, but recognize that you are not a therapist.

The first lesson promotes an understanding of the problem of youth suicide. Students are asked a number of questions to stimulate their thinking and to clarify the many misperceptions that exist. Students are also asked to identify community resources to assist suicidal youths. Students are asked to visit such agencies and to gather information about them.

The second lesson emphasizes the warning signs and stresses that depression is common and situational in nature. An activity is provided that encourages students to think about a time when they were depressed. The exercise focuses on how they felt and acted at that time, to whom they talked, and what helped them through the depressed period.

The third lesson centers on stress, substance use, and suicide risk. The variety of stressors that teenagers face are emphasized. The relationship between stress and drug/alcohol usage is emphasized. Positive steps to cope with stress are emphasized.

The goal of the fourth lesson is to help students communicate with and assist a suicidal friend. It is pointed out that secrets must not be kept about suicidal behavior. Activities are provided for students to practice and discuss communication skills. Steps in helping a suicidal friend are identified. Because students often try to solve the problem of a suicidal person rather than focusing on the person's feelings, students are encouraged to role-play a number of scenarios where one student responds to a suicidal friend. In these role plays, showing caring, providing empathetic responses, giving support, and lending perspective are emphasized.

The final lesson focuses on help available in the community. Students are asked to share their reports on the community agencies that they contacted as part of the homework for the first lesson. A master list of community services is made for each student. An activity is also provided to demonstrate locating help in an emergency. It is suggested that students receive a wallet-size card with community resource information on it. The one component that seems to be missing from the resource list is services at school. It would seem beneficial to include that as an immediate and available source of help, and to emphasize adults in general, especially parents.

Each lesson provides goals and objectives, preparation suggestions, handouts ready for duplicating, and possible homework assignments. A number of role-play scenarios are also provided.

The Samaritans Program

As noted earlier, the Samaritans, an international organization for suicide prevention, has published a manual for teachers (Fencik, 1986). The manual is based on the premise that education about suicide and its warning signs will save lives. The role of the schools in assisting with the social problem of youth suicide is stressed. The manual is divided into five lessons to be conducted in the classroom. Each lesson requires at least one period. Teachers are given the option of picking and choosing from the five lessons, with the exception that the third lesson, on the warning signs of suicide, must be included. It is also left up to teachers whether or not to administer the 18-item test on suicide and whether or not to use the various handouts. The Samaritans manual has two basic goals: first, to raise school personnel's awareness of youth suicide and to show them how to intervene to assist a suicidal student; second, to provide teenagers with other options besides suicide to deal with their problems.

The first lesson emphasizes developing a compassionate attitude toward suicide and its victims. Students are provided with open-ended statements to explore their attitudes toward suicide. The teacher should emphasize that there are no right or wrong answers. Either an entire-classroom discussion or a small-group discussion of attitudes is acceptable. The manual states, "The teacher should be sensitive to and understanding of the variety of expressed attitudes. Allow the students to possess their attitudes. To stifle them would close off the possibility of growth and change (Fencik, 1986, p. 12).

The second lesson stresses acquiring knowledge about suicide. This lesson points out that many myths exist about suicide, and much fear results from all the misunderstandings and misperceptions. Students need to know the truth about suicide. Students are asked to respond to 18 true-or-false questions about suicide. The students keep their questionnaires, and then the teacher goes over each item and gives the students correct information. Students are also given handouts on frequently asked questions and on myths and facts about suicide.

The third lesson, on the warning signs of suicide, is the one required lesson. Its objectives are to inform students about the warning signs, to clarify causation factors, and to convince students that adult help is necessary to save a friend or oneself from suicide. Students are provided with a handout on the causes of teen suicide, as well as with a list of verbal, behavioral, and situational warning signs.

The fourth lesson emphasizes teaching the students "befriending" skills. A poem is provided that points out the importance of really listening to others and not being too quick to give advice. Several objectives are identified to increase students' ability to befriend others. Befriending is defined as friendship characterized by the following:

- Being nonjudgmental and humble.
- Being compassionate and available.
- Sharing the person's pain and reflecting his or her feelings.
- Listening instead of giving advice.
- Maintaining confidentiality except when suicidal ideation is involved.
- Providing acceptance, empathy, and caring.

Two students also role-play a situation in which one student is suicidal. The class then discusses the role play and decides whether or not the befriender utilized the recommended skills. Students also are asked to write a short essay on this topic: "What is listening as practiced by a befriender?"

The final lesson focuses on the support system and ways in which to assist a suicidal student. It is emphasized that suicidal persons do want to be rescued and do not truly want to die. Instead, they want things to get better and need support. The teacher and befriending students can be an integral part of the support system. A support system flow chart is provided that shows the following referral steps:

1. Trained students and staff befriend a troubled student.
2. Suicidal students are identified.
3. Suicidal students receive support services, both within the school and within the community.
4. Befriending continues, both in and out of school.

Several fictional examples are provided to sharpen befriending skills and to illustrate referral procedures.

PRESENTATIONS IN ONE CLASS PERIOD

What should the teacher include if he or she has one class period to devote to suicide prevention? The California State Department of Education (1987) recommends that the following key points should be emphasized:

- Warning signs
- How to cope with stress
- Communicating with a suicidal friend and getting help for him or her

I believe that two additional points should also be emphasized: (1) the situational nature of suicide, and (2) the fact that substance use makes things worse, not better. Students should also be allowed to ask any questions that they have on the subject, and an example of successful intervention by a friend should be provided.

Should a teacher take most of the one class period to show a film on suicide prevention? I recommend that this not be done, although it would be the easiest way for a teacher to present a 1-day unit. There needs to be a good deal of interaction between the teacher and the students, and showing a film may take too much time and not allow for discussion.

ROLE PLAYS

Several of the curriculum programs emphasize the importance of having students role-play. The purposes of role plays are twofold: first, to have students practice listening and befriending skills; second, to have students practice intervening with a friend and notifying an adult about suicidal ideation. The California State Department of Education (1987) makes a number of recommendations about the use of role plays. The teacher should set the scene and suggest key points for the class to focus on. In addition, students should distance themselves personally from their roles, and props should be used to help the role player separate himself or herself from the role being played. After the role-play experience, the participants should be asked questions about their experience and how they felt at various points. A classroom discussion should be held that emphasizes the purpose of the dramatization, feelings and insights that the students had, and conclusions that they reach about the exercise and problem solving. The students who participated in the role play should be called by their real names before the period is over. A student should not be forced to role-play a suicidal teenager.

INFORMATION FOR FACULTY

Should the information presented to school personnel be substantially different from the information presented to students? No. Everyone needs the same basic information about the warning signs and ways to respond to them. Everyone must know the referral process and sources of help. The California State Department of Education (1987) uses the same handouts for both students and faculty. The faculty does need additional information about ethical and liability issues.

INFORMATION FOR PARENTS

Parents should receive the same basic information that students and teachers receive. The school district's procedures and help available at school should be clarified. Parents need to be aware that suicide may be on their children's minds, and they need to know what to look for and to understand that direct inquiry is needed. Information can be presented to parents through evening presentations and through district newsletters.

Lennox (1987) lists the following areas that should be emphasized to parents:

- Communication and sharing with their children
- Skills of parenting and setting limits
- Signs and symptoms of stress
- Characteristics of drug/alcohol abuse
- Building children's self-esteem

USE OF FILMS

Does showing a film on suicide prevention help students master the objectives? Several of the curriculum programs reviewed above make use of films and others do not. Students today are very visually oriented, and films are often used to complement lecture presentations. I have found that educational films such as those recommended earlier in this book (*Young People in Crisis, Suicide—The Warning Signs,* and *Teens Who Choose Life*) help students grasp key points about suicide prevention. A film can illustrate a suicidal person's ambivalence—throwing away pills and then searching for them—much more effectively than a lecture! Films also dramatically illustrate friend intervention and empower students with the awareness that they, too, could save a life!

WHEN SURVIVORS PARTICIPATE IN PRESENTATIONS

One possible situation school personnel should look out for is that of having a survivor of a family suicide present in a class in which suicide prevention is discussed. This situation requires special planning, as survivors can be more sensitive to certain issues than other students. As one survivor commented to me, "The discussion of suicide caught me off guard; my teacher didn't warn me and I felt uncomfortable. She alluded to the suicide of my brother last year but didn't make it clear. Some members of the class knew about it but not everyone." A second survivor was offended because the discussion focused on the suicide of his brother. He said, "I can't believe it but the teacher asked me to bring his suicide note in and let the class see it. That's going too far! I refused to bring in the note."

Offending or hurting the survivor can be avoided by doing the following:

1. Prepare the survivors for the curriculum unit in advance and give them the option of participating in it.
2. Acknowledge in a compassionate way the suicide of their loved one but do not dwell on the details. Instead, focus on prevention of future suicides.

SUMMARY

Curriculum presentations on suicide prevention are needed to raise awareness both in the schools and in the community. Such presentations in the schools are almost always the result of a school's having experienced one or more suicides. Ideally, a unit on suicide prevention would take several class periods and be part of an overall mental health unit.

Suicide prevention needs to be introduced in junior high, or at least by the first year of high school. The emphasis should be on recognizing the warning signs and intervening to save a life. These skills are not just needed in the teen years, but are needed throughout adulthood as well.

There are those who argue that suicide should not be discussed, because the idea of suicide will be planted thereby in someone's mind. Historically, there has been a reluctance to discuss it, as well as to show compassion to those who think about it or to those who are victims or survivors. The incidence of youth suicide and the surveys showing that it is on the minds of today's youths necessitate that we give them accurate information about it and how they can help one another. Carefully planned curriculum units can do much to reduce the number of youth suicides.

11

Questions and Answers

Q. *How should the school respond to media requests for interviews after a suicide?*

A. Schools should anticipate being in this position and prepare in advance. A cooperative approach is recommended. The media can do much to minimize contagion factors.

Q. *Has any national legislation on suicide prevention been passed?*

A. No. A number of bills have been proposed, but none have passed. Conservative groups have labeled such legislation "death education."

Q. *Who at school should be told that a student is suicidal?*

A. It is recommended that everyone who directly supervises the student should be told. Personnel who do not directly supervise the student but who need to know are the principal and counselor.

Q. *Have schools been sued for having an inadequate suicide prevention program?*

A. Yes. Schools have been found to be liable for negligence when they failed to adequately supervise students who were known to be suicidal. The key point is whether or not the school personnel could "foresee" the suicide attempt.

Q. *Does almost everyone at least think of suicide during his or her lifetime?*

A. Yes. Everyone gives it some thought.

Q. *Is there a certain time of the year when more suicides occur—for example, at holiday times?*

A. No. There is a slight increase in the spring, but there is no one time of the year, such as Christmas, when a disproportionate number of suicides occur.

Q. *Which states have passed suicide prevention legislation?*
A. At this writing, Alabama, California, Florida, New Jersey, Texas, and Wisconsin.

Q. *Don't students have a right to kill themselves if they really want to?*
A. No. Students who are suicidal are planning a permanent solution to a temporary problem. Everyone must recognize that adolescents do not truly want to die and respond to intervention.

Q. *Do losses of loved ones or relationships have much to do with youth suicide?*
A. Yes. Students who have experienced numerous losses may feel helpless and hopeless and turn to suicide. We also must take the breakup of adolescent romances seriously, because such breakups often precipitate suicide attempts.

Q. *Will teenagers talk about their suicidal thoughts?*
A. Yes, if they are provided with an opportunity to do so by someone they trust. The key is to let them talk and reflect their feelings. Their suicidal thoughts should not be dismissed or minimized.

Q. *Is suicide a leading cause of death in the United States?*
A. Yes. It is the seventh leading cause of death across all ages. It is the second leading cause of death for teenagers.

Q. *What methods do adolescents use most often to commit suicide?*
A. Guns account for approximately 60% of adolescent suicides. Gun safety programs and convincing families not to have guns accessible in the home are keys to prevention.

Q. *Do males attempt suicide more often than females?*
A. No, females attempt more often than males. Males complete suicide more often because they use more lethal methods.

Q. *Can schools plant suicide in the minds of students by discussing it?*
A. No. Adolescents are very much aware of youth suicide as a societal problem. By *not* talking about it, schools allow misperceptions to interfere with students' being helped.

Q. *Can students who talk about suicide be classified as low-risk?*
A. No. Students who talk about it are at risk. If they do not receive prompt attention, they may act out their suicidal thoughts.

Q. *Are teenagers who commit suicide mentally ill?*
A. No, most are not. They are overwhelmed by problems and losses in their lives and have not developed adequate coping skills.

Q. *Has the rate of youth suicide really increased that much, or is it just being publicized more widely?*

A. The rate has increased 300% since the 1950s.

Q. *What is the role of the school?*

A. To detect suicidal behavior, assess the severity level of students' symptoms, notify parents, and secure the needed services and supervision for students.

Q. *When should curriculum presentations on suicide prevention begin?*

A. Most experts recommend beginning to give some information in junior high, and beginning a concentrated curriculum program in ninth grade.

Q. *How do suicidal students react when they are told that their parents must be notified?*

A. Most react cooperatively and are actually relieved that their parents are going to know how troubled they are. Some students will express concern at the anticipated reactions of their parents. The student needs reassurance that the counselor will elicit a supportive reaction from their parents.

Q. *How far should school personnel go to try to stop a suicide by a student?*

A. Schools should take every step possible. This might mean physically detaining a student known to be suicidal.

Q. *Will it be costly to work on suicide prevention in the schools?*

A. No. Most schools already have personnel who could be trained at little or no cost. The issue is one of recognizing the problem and accepting responsibility.

Q. *What should the qualifications be for someone who counsels school children about suicide?*

A. I believe that knowledge about suicide and about how to assist a suicidal person is more important than whether the person has a particular degree or credential.

Q. *How can we determine the youth suicide rate in our city or state in comparison to the national trends?*

A. Some cities do not keep accurate records. There may be a city or county office with statistics. The CDC publishes incidence figures by state (see CDC, 1986).

Q. *What can the school do when a suicidal adolescent is released from the hospital?*

A. Communicate with hospital treatment personnel prior to the return to school, and meet with the adolescent on his or her return to discuss support. At this time, have the adolescent sign a "no-suicide" contract. Monitor the adolescent closely; if he or she appears to be contemplating another suicide attempt, notify the parents and recommend outpatient therapy or rehospitalization.

Q. *Is there an assessment scale that can indicate without a doubt whether a student is suicidal?*

A. No. A careful history of the adolescent's coping pattern and current stressors, and an analysis of his or her suicidal thoughts and plans, are needed.

Q. *Are no-suicide contracts effective in preventing youth suicide?*

A. Yes. No-suicide contracts help adolescents to take control of their suicidal thoughts and give the adolescents sources of help when the suicidal thoughts return.

Q. *How can we obtain administrative support to implement a suicide intervention program?*

A. Gather data about youth suicide and its incidence. Provide administrators with samples of school intervention programs. Stress the need to clarify the district's responsibility in this area. Be persistent, draw up procedures, and submit them for administrative approval.

Q. *Is there a single cause or reason to explain teen suicide?*

A. No. Researchers have identified as many as 28 causes, and each individual is unique.

Q. *Is there a certain type of student who is at risk for suicide?*

A. No, there is no one type. Depression has long been associated with youth suicide. Recently, emphasis has also been placed on conduct disorders and substance use as associated problems.

Q. *How can schools help survivors?*

A. Close contact should be maintained with surviving students and their parents. Outside counseling and participation in survivor groups should be encouraged.

Q. *How should I respond to a suicidal student?*

A. Respond openly, honestly, and directly. Let the student know that you care. Give him or her permission to talk about suicidal thoughts.

Stay with the student, explain the referral procedures, and emphasize that help is available.

Q. *Is suicide a crime?*
A. No. It used to be a crime, but for all practical purpose it is not a crime to attempt or commit suicide.

Q. *Is a large school assembly a good setting for discussing the suicide of a student?*
A. No. We do not want to glorify or sensationalize a death by suicide in any way. A small-group or homeroom discussion is recommended.

Q. *Why do drugs and alcohol play such a large role in youth suicide?*
A. Drugs and alcohol impair contact with reality and contribute to a teenager's acting on suicidal thoughts. Alcohol and drugs are also depressants and make young people further depressed.

Q. *How can youth suicide be detected?*
A. Careful attention must be paid to the verbal and behavioral warning signs that young people give approximately 90% of the time.

Q. *Why do young people talk about their suicidal thoughts and plans?*
A. They are asking for help. They go back and forth between wanting to live and wanting to die. More than anything, they want their lives to change.

Q. *Can the suicide of one adolescent "trigger" the suicide of another?*
A. Yes. Adolescents are more likely to imitate the suicide of another than adults are. Factors believed to be involved are impulsivity, impressionability, and striving for recognition or glamorization through suicidal actions.

Q. *Where does the responsibility of the school end when a student is detected as suicidal?*
A. Responsibility lessens when parents are notified and community services are obtained. School personnel should continue to monitor the student as long as he or she attends school.

Q. *Could the content of a student's artwork or poetry be a sign that the student is thinking of suicide?*
A. Yes. The content and meaning of both poetry and artwork should be examined closely. The teacher may need to inquire directly about whether or not the student has had suicidal thoughts. If this is the case, then school referral procedures should be followed.

Q. *May a student who runs away be at risk for suicide?*

A. Yes. Research has shown that from 20% to 25% of adolescents who run away attempt suicide.

Q. *Will adolescents who are prevented from killing themselves once keep trying until they succeed?*

A. No. Most suicide attempts are situational in nature. The adolescent who is stopped and who gets professional help is unlikely to try again.

12

Resources

THE AMERICAN ASSOCIATION OF SUICIDOLOGY

The AAS has much information to offer the public schools. The organization is composed of many professionals who share a common interest in suicide prevention. Colt (1986) has commented, "There is no federally funded research on suicide; organized efforts in prevention rest largely with AAS" (p. 37). Colt also points out that there have been conflicts in the organization between mental health professionals and crisis center volunteers. These conflicts have resulted in some feeling that the AAS has too much of a lay orientation.

Johnson and Maile (1987) point out several valuable activities of the AAS: sponsoring a large national convention each year, distributing a monthly newsletter entitled *Newslink*, and certifying crisis hotlines. Members of the organization also receive the quarterly publication *Suicide and Life-Threatening Behavior*. In addition, the AAS publishes a number of brochures and handouts on suicide prevention, as well as a directory of survivor groups and crisis centers in the United States.

Johnson and Maile (1987) suggest that a representative of the school district join the AAS and attend the national convention to gather information. Individuals may join for $75 a year, and institutional dues are $150. The AAS has shown much interest in recent years in the schools. The organization has a School Program Committee with the following subcommittees: Training and Resources; Legislative; Funding; Research and Evaluation; Standards and Guidelines; and Communication. The AAS may be contacted at 2459 South Ash, Denver, CO 80222. The phone number is (303) 692-0985.

OTHER NATIONAL INFORMATION SOURCES

National Committee on Youth Suicide Prevention
665 5th Avenue, 13th Floor
New York, NY 10103
(212) 957-9292

Suicide Research Unit
National Institute of Mental Health
5600 Fishers Lane
Rockville, MD 20857

Youth Suicide National Center, East Coast Office
1825 I Street N.W., Suite 945
Washington, DC 20006
(202) 429-2016

Youth Suicide National Center, West Coast Office
1811 Trousdale Drive
Burlingame, CA 94010
(414) 877-5604

The Youth Suicide National Center provides an extensive list of resources, including pamphlets, brochures, article reprints, and recommended films and books for both teens and professionals. The *Report of
the National Conference on Youth Suicide,* held in 1985, is also available
from the center.

Office of the Inspector General
U.S. Department of Health and Human Services
2901 Third Avenue, MS 309
Seattle, WA 98121
(206) 442-0491

The OIG is the publisher of *Youth Suicide National Program Inspection*
(1986), which gives information about initiatives from every state.

Centers for Disease Control
U.S. Department of Health and Human Services
1600 Clifton Road, N.E.
Atlanta, GA 30333

The CDC is the publisher of *Youth Suicide in the United States, 1970 to
1980* (1986).

Suicide Information and Education Center
#201 1615 10th Avenue, S.W.
Calgary, Alberta T3C 0J7, Canada
(403) 245-3900

The Suicide Information and Education Center serves as a data base, resource center, and information clearinghouse. The center has a com-
puter-based storage and retrieval system with over 8,000 citations. It also
publishes several journals and runs a newspaper clipping service.

National Coalition on Television Violence
P.O. Box 2157
Champaign, IL 61820

The coalition publishes newsletters that contain information about
drugs, violence, and suicide portrayal on television.

PUBLISHERS OF BOOKS ON SUICIDE

Guilford Press
72 Spring Street
New York, NY 10012

Springer Publishing Company
200 Park Avenue South
New York, NY 10003

Charles C Thomas, Publisher
2600 South First Street
Springfield, IL 62794

The Center for Thanatology Research and Education, Inc.
391 Atlantic Avenue
Brooklyn, NY 11217

Learning Publications, Inc.
P.O. Box 1326
Holmes Beach, FL 34218
(813) 778-6818

This publisher sponsored the first national conference on Suicide Prevention and the Schools in Florida in 1987. It also publishes a quarterly
newsletter entitled *School Intervention Report*.

SCHOOL PROGRAM GUIDES

Suicide Prevention: A Resource and Planning Guide
Publication Sales Office
Wisconsin Department of Instruction
125 S. Webster Street
P.O. Box 7641
Madison, WI 53707 $8.00

The Adolescent Suicide Prevention Program
Fairfax County Schools
Belle Willard Ad Center
10310 Layton Hall Drive
Fairfax, VA 22030 $3.00

A School Approach for the Prevention of Youth Suicide
Indiana State Board of Health
1330 W. Michigan St., Room 203
Indianapolis, IN 46206-1964   Free

Suicide Prevention Program for the California Public Schools
California State Department of Education
P.O. Box 271
Sacramento, CA 95802-0271 $8.48

Handbook: Suicide Prevention in the Schools, by S. Ruof, J. Harris,
and M. Robbie
Special Education
Weld Boces
P.O. Box 578
LaSalle, CO 80645 $12.50

Suicide Intervention and Prevention, by S. Lindborg and N. Wagner
Minnesota School Psychology Association
Monograph No. 2
Attention: Andrea Canter
4438 Pillsbury Avenue South
Minneapolis, MN 55409 $5.00

Adolescent Suicide Awareness Program Manual: A Comprehensive Education and Prevention Program for School Communities
South Bergen Mental Health Center, Inc.
646 B Valley Brook Avenue
Lyndhurst, NJ 07071 $7.00

JOURNALS

Suicide and Life-Threatening Behavior (official journal of the AAS)
Guilford Press
72 Spring Street
New York, NY 10012
    Individuals $32.00
    Institutions $90.00

Suicide Research Digest
Center for Suicide Research and Prevention
Rush–Presbyterian–St. Luke's Medical Center
1720 West Polk Street
Chicago, IL 60612
    Individuals $30.00 (2-year subscription)
    Institutions $45.00

BOOKS ON THE SCHOOL'S ROLE
IN SUICIDE PREVENTION

Barrett, T. (1985). *Youth in Crisis: Seeking Solutions to Self-Destructive Behavior*
Sopris West, Inc.
1120 Delaware Avenue
Longmont, CO 80501

Johnson, S., and Maile, L. (1987). *Suicide and the Schools*
Charles C Thomas, Publisher
2600 South First Street
Springfield, IL 62794

Guetzloe, E. (in press). *Youth Suicide: What the Educator Should Know*
The Council for Exceptional Children
1920 Association Drive
Reston, VA 22091

CURRICULUM GUIDES

A Teacher's Manual for the Prevention of Suicide among Adolescents,
edited by J. Fencik
The Samaritans, Inc.
33 Chestnut Street
Providence, RI 02093
(401) 272-4044 $10.00

Smith, J. (1988). *A Crisis Intervention Curriculum for Teenagers and
Young Adults*
Learning Publications, Inc.
P.O. Box 1326
Holmes Beach, FL 34218 $14.95

Lifelines: Sequential Curricula on Adolescent Suicide, by M. Underwood,
C. Jakubik, and J. Kalafat
Department of Consultation and Education
St. Clare's Hospital
Denville, NJ 07834
(201) 625-7080

FILM AND MEDIA RESOURCES

Youth Suicide National Center
See "Other National Information Sources," above

The center publishes a reviewed list of 33 films and media resources.

Telemedia Publishing Inc.
50 Holly Street
Toronto, Ontario M4S 3B3, Canada
(416) 482-8600

Guidance Associates
Communications Park
P.O. Box 3000
Mount Kisco, NY 10549-0900
(800) 431-2266

Sunburst Communications
101 Castleton Street
Pleasantville, NY 10570-9971
(800) 431-1934

Exar Communications, Inc.
Distributions Operations
267B McClean Avenue
Staten Island, NY 10305
(718) 720-4488

Coronet Films
420 Academy Drive
Northbrook, IL 60062
(718) 940-1260

13

Conclusions

This book has been written to clarify the many questions that exist about the role of the schools with regard to suicide intervention. I have been fortunate to have a large staff of psychologists, as well as excellent administrative support that has made crisis intervention the top priority for the psychological services staff. Lindborg and Wagner (1987) have referred to the program that I direct as the "Cadillac Model." Although not every school district may have these advantages, every district, regardless of size, should have a suicide intervention program with written policies that are understood by all who work in the district.

There has been a dramatic increase in the number of youth suicides. School administrators have been slow to acknowledge this increase, to accept responsibility, and to devote resources to do something about it. In particular, administrators have used the debate about whether or not curriculum awareness programs encourage youth suicide as a reason not to formalize a program. A debate does exist as to the advisability of curriculum awareness programs; however, I know of no mental health professionals or suicidologists who do not support teaching school staff members the warning signs of suicide, training counselors to assist suicidal students, and developing prevention and postvention policies.

The role of the school is to detect suicidal students, assess the severity level of their suicidal thoughts or actions, notify their parents, and secure needed supervision and services for them. The three-level crisis intervention model developed by Caplan (1964) has been used in this book to demonstrate a way in which schools can organize their efforts. Suicide prevention programs in the schools began in California in the 1970s and have spread to approximately 125 to 200 school systems at this writing. There is no way to know for sure how many schools have a program. The fact that each system has been left to its own devices to struggle with this problem has been pointed out by Tugend (1984).

This book is an attempt to provide practical information so that each school district does not have to reinvent the wheel. Legislation to require school districts to have suicide intervention programs has been passed by six states, and proposals have at least been raised in a number of other states. Federal legislation, which is sorely needed, has been proposed on numerous occasions but has not been passed.

Youth suicide is a societal problem with many causative factors; at least 28 different factors have been identified. Recently, school districts that have inadequately supervised suicidal students have been sued and have been found liable. By contrast, no school districts have been sued for having a prevention program. Incidence figures have shown that as many as 10% of high school students make attempts and as many as 40–60% consider suicide.

It has been pointed out that teachers are the logical personnel to identify suicidal students. Teachers are in a key position; however, I recommend that all support personnel, including aides, bus drivers, and cafeteria workers, receive in-service training on suicide. Some have questioned how much responsibility should be placed on teachers. The California State Department of Education (1987) emphasizes that educators have a responsibility to protect the health and safety of students.

Many misperceptions still exist about youth suicide, and one of the goals of a prevention program should be to give school personnel the facts and to empower them with the awareness that they can save a life. Two key myths that still persist are, first, that the young person who talks about suicide will not commit suicide; and, second, that once a person is suicidal he or she is always suicidal.

The aftermath of a student suicide is very difficult for a school system. Prior planning is essential to help the survivors at school. Postvention activities actually prevent further suicides.

There is a pressing need for more research about youth suicide. I agree with Ryerson (1988), who has called for a collaborative effort between researchers and program personnel. I cannot agree with Shaffer (1988), who has called for a moratorium on suicide curriculum awareness programs. There are simply too many teenagers out there struggling with questions about their own existence or that of their friends. Teenagers need to know the facts about suicide, how to prevent it, and how to solve problems.

No immediate decline is expected in the youth suicide rate. Suicide must be addressed as a serious health problem in this country. What better place to start prevention efforts than with our young people? It is important to arm them with the skills to identify and help suicidal individuals.

I was not prepared for the reality of youth suicide when I began working in the public schools. The problem does exist, and school personnel are struggling with it on their own; they want desperately to help but are not sure how. Suicide prevention is everyone's responsibility. Every school district needs a comprehensive suicide intervention program that is coordinated with community resources.

Appendices

APPENDIX A. TEENAGE SUICIDE PREVENTION TIPS

The tragic dilemma of youths wanting to take their own lives is one we don't expect to go away any time soon. We believe that one of the most important curative factors is open and direct communication. Sometimes this necessitates reporting information given in confidence in order to save a life. We also are convinced that students are often in a better position to help other students. Let us encourage our students to look out for each other and to seek help for a friend if that friend won't seek it out on his or her own.

As the school personnel most directly involved with students on a daily basis, your observations and feelings are important to those of us who provide psychological services. We are enormously proud of your efforts over the past few years in keeping us informed concerning students you were worried about.

Listed below is a brief summary of clues to potential suicide, as well as some suggestions for how you can help.

What to Look For

1. *Verbal signs*: "I wish I were dead," "No one cares whether I live or die," "Things would be better if I weren't here."

2. *Behavioral clues*: Alcohol or drug abuse, previous attempts, giving away possessions, making a will, sudden change in behavior (e.g., quiet student becomes talkative, friendly student becomes quiet), significant drop in grades, risk-taking behavior resulting in accidents or injuries.

From *Teenage Prevention Suicide Tips* by R. Schindler and S. Poland, 1985, unpublished manuscript, Cypress–Fairbanks Independent School District, Cypress, TX. Reprinted by permission of the authors and the Cypress–Fairbanks Independent School District.

3. *Situational cues*: end of a serious relationship, divorce or death of a parent, family financial difficulties, moving to new location (or other stresses among family members).

4. *Syndromatic clues*: social isolation, depression, disorientation, changes in sleeping and/or eating patterns, dissatisfaction (i.e., constant complaining, help-less–hopeless feelings).

How You Can Help

Step 1: Listen and hear. Of vital importance to a person in an emotional crisis is to have available someone who will listen and hear what he or she is saying. Avoid false reassurances that "everything will be okay," and never demean suicidal expressions. Don't be judgmental or moralizing.

Step 2: Be supportive. Communicate your concern for the person.

Step 3: Be sensitive to the relative seriousness of the thoughts and feelings. Inquire directly about thoughts of suicide. If we don't respond to students' suicidal thoughts, they may interpret our reaction as not caring. Suicide is a topic that makes us all uncomfortable, but we must face it with open, honest communication. When a person speaks of clear-cut self-destructive plans, the situation is usually much more serious. *Take any suicidal complaint seriously, even if expressed in a calm voice.*

Step 4: Trust your own judgment. If you believe someone is in danger of suicide, act on your beliefs. Don't let others mislead you into ignoring suicide signals. *Be an alarmist.*

Step 5: Act definitively.

   A. *Tell others.* Share your knowledge with the counselor and/or school psychologist. Don't worry about breaking a confidence. You may have to betray a secret to save a life.

   B. *Stay with a suicidal person.* Don't leave a suicidal person alone if you think there is immediate danger. Stay with the person until help arrives. Call upon whoever is needed; do not try to handle everything alone.

Step 6: Be aware of previous attempts. A student who has made a previous attempt is at high risk to try again. *If you are aware that a student has made a previous attempt, tell the counselor and/or the school psychologist.* Make sure they know.

What Happens after the Teacher Alerts the Counselor and/or School Psychologist?

The counselor and/or school psychologist will utilize their expertise to assess the lethality risk of the student's suicidal ideation. The parents of the student will be contacted, and we will work with them to increase the supervision of the student and help the family gain the needed intervention. This intervention would probably involve counseling outside of the public school and possibly even hospitalization. Feedback about the severity of the situation, as well as how you as a teacher can help, will be provided as much as is professionally reasonable.

APPENDIX B. SUICIDE INFORMATION TEST

True/false

_____ 1. The incidence of teenage suicide has increased almost 300% since the 1950s.

_____ 2. Teenagers who make plans to commit suicide keep their thoughts to themselves, and the suicide occurs without warning.

_____ 3. Suicidal teenagers are fully intent on dying.

_____ 4. A person who is suicidal will always be suicidal.

_____ 5. There is no relationship between drugs/alcohol and suicide.

_____ 6. There are one or two causes or motives that explain most suicides.

_____ 7. Suicidal tendencies are inherited, and suicide runs in families.

_____ 8. Teenagers who threaten suicide and make suicidal gestures are attempting to manipulate others and should be ignored.

_____ 9. There is a certain type of person who commits suicide.

_____ 10. Suicide is always the act of a mentally ill or psychotic person.

_____ 11. Talking openly about suicide may cause a suicidal person to commit suicide.

_____ 12. Improvement following a suicidal crisis means that there is no more chance of suicide.

_____ 13. Everyone who commits suicide is depressed.

_____ 14. Removing the means of suicide (e.g., removal of handguns and poisons) would prevent many suicides.

_____ 15. Deaths by firearms account for most suicides.

_____ 16. There is a particular time of year that most suicides occur.

_____ 17. There are over 100 attempts for every completed suicide.

_____ 18. Young children never commit suicide.

_____ 19. Suicide is the second leading cause of death among adolescents.

_____ 20. Suicidal adolescents will be angry at those who attempt to stop them from committing suicide.

_____ 21. The religious belief that suicide is wrong will prevent someone from committing suicide.

_____ 22. Most suicides occur at home between the hours of 3 P.M. and midnight.

_____ 23. Surveys have shown that as many as 8–10 of every 100 adolescents have attempted suicide.

_____ 24. Teenagers who are suicidal will tell adults instead of their friends about their suicidal thoughts or actions.

_____ 25. Suicide is only a problem among teenagers.

_____ 26. Females make more suicide attempts than males and use less lethal means.

_____ 27. Males and females are becoming more alike in method and completion of suicide.

_____ 28. Each person has a right to commit suicide, and it is wrong to intervene.

APPENDIX C. SUICIDE INFORMATION TEST ANSWERS

1. True.

2. False. Approximately 90% give some kind of verbal or behavioral warning.

3. False. Most teenagers are ambivalent about their death, and more than anything want something to change to end the pain they are experiencing.

4. False. Suicide is situational in nature. A person who receives help and is prevented from attempting suicide may never try again.

5. False. Drugs and/or alcohol are involved with the majority of youth suicides. Drugs and alcohol reduce normal inhibitions against suicide.

6. False. There are many causes of youth suicide, with each individual having a unique set of circumstances in his or her life history.

7. False. There is no evidence that suicide is inherited, although a predisposition to depression may be inherited. A history of suicide in the family does increase the risk but does not make it inevitable.

8. False. Threats and attempts should be taken seriously and as the teenagers' pleas for help.

9. False. Suicide occurs across all classes and with all types of people.

10. False. The person who commits suicide is unhappy but not necessarily mentally ill. The suicide may be the result of many life stresses and losses that the person could not cope with. The person may be rational and in touch with reality.

11. False. We must inquire directly and deal openly with this topic, and by doing so we provide the support and assistance that a suicidal person needs.

12. False. People who have been suicidal need continuing assistance. Individuals who have been extremely depressed may not have enough energy to carry out their suicidal plans and need to be monitored closely as their extreme depression lifts.

13. False. Depression alone does not account for all suicides. There is increasing evidence that adolescents with conduct and substance abuse problems are also at risk.

14. True. Many experts believe the single best way to prevent a suicide is to remove the lethal means.

15. True. Firearms account for approximately 60% of all suicides.

16. False. There is no clear-cut evidence that suicides are higher at certain holidays or seasons of the year.

17. True. Estimates range from 50 to 120 attempts for each completed suicide.

18. False. Suicide is rare under the age of 14, but it does happen. Children are likely to engage in risk-taking behavior.

19. True. According to Leder (1987), suicide is the second leading cause of death among teenagers, with accidents being the leading cause of death.

20. False. They may be initially angry, but mostly are relieved that someone cares enough to help them.

21. False. They may believe that suicide is wrong, but see no other alternative to end their pain.

22. True. It is believed that suicidal people pick a time to commit suicide when someone is there who could stop them.

23. True.

24. False. Studies have shown that as much as 90% of the time, teenagers tell their friends first, and they do not always tell adults.

25. False. Suicide must be addressed as a societal problem across all ages. The rate for young adults (19–24) is higher than that for teenagers. The suicide rate then declines after age 24, but increases for the middle-aged and elderly.

26. True. Females make suicide attempts three to four times as often as males, and have traditionally used less lethal methods, such as pills and wrist cutting.

27. True. Females are increasingly using more lethal means, such as firearms.

28. False. Suicidal people do not truly want to die, and we have a moral and ethical responsibility to intervene.

APPENDIX D. SUICIDE RISK ASSESSMENT WORKSHEET

Instructions: Use as a checklist and average for final assessment. Each item carries the same weight.

Probability of Attempt: Low __ Medium __ High __

	Risk present, but lower	Medium	Higher
1. Suicide plan			
A. Details	— Vague	— Some specifics	— Well thought out; knows when, where, how
B. Availability of means	— Not available, will have to get	— Available, has close by	— Has in hand
C. Time	— No specific time or in future	— Within a few hours	— Immediately
D. Lethality of method	— Pills, slash wrists	— Drugs and alcohol, car wreck, carbon monoxide	— Gun, hanging, jumping
E. Chance of intervention	— Others present most of the time	— Others available if called upon	— No one nearby; isolated
2. Previous suicide attempts	— None or one of low lethality	— Multiple of low lethality or one of medium lethality; history of repeated threats	— One of high lethality or multiple of moderate
3. Stress	— No significant stress	— Moderate reaction to loss and environmental changes	— Severe reaction to loss or environmental changes
4. Symptoms			
A. Coping behavior	— Daily activities continue as usual with little change	— Some daily activities disrupted; disturbance in eating, sleeping, school work	— Gross disturbances in daily functioning
B. Depression	— Mild; feels slightly down	— Moderate; some moodiness, sadness, irritability, loneliness, and decrease of energy	— Overwhelmed with hopelessness, sadness, and feelings of worthlessness
5. Resources	— Help available; significant others concerned and willing to help	— Family and friends available but unwilling to help consistently	— Family and friends not available or hostile, exhausted, injurious
6. Communication aspects	— Direct expression of feelings and suicidal intent	— Interpersonalized suicidal goal ("They'll be sorry—I'll show them")	— Very indirect or nonverbal expression of internalized suicidal goal (guilt, worthlessness)
7. Life style	— Stable relationships, personality, and school performance	— Recent acting-out behavior and substance abuse; acute suicidal behavior in stable personality	— Suicidal behavior in unstable personality; emotional disturbance; repeated difficulty with peers, family, and teachers
8. Medical status	— No significant medical problems	— Acute but short-term or psychosomatic illness	— Chronic debilitating or acute catastrophic illness

Total checks:	— Low	— Medium	— High

Student name _____ I.D. # _____ Date _____ Counselor _____

From *Suicide Risk Assessment Worksheet* by J. Smith, 1988a, unpublished manuscript, Dallas Independent School District, Dallas, TX. Reprinted by permission of the author and the Dallas Independent School District.

APPENDIX E. VERIFICATION OF EMERGENCY CONFERENCE

I, or we, _____, the parents of _____, were involved in a conference with school personnel on _____. We have been notified that our child is suicidal. We have been further advised that we should seek some psychological/ psychiatric consultation immediately from the community. We have been provided with a list of community services. The school district has clarified its role and will provide follow-up assistance to our child to support the treatment services from the community.

_____

Parent or Legal Guardian

_____

Parent or Legal Guardian

_____

School Staff Member Title

_____

School Staff Member Title

References

American Association of Suicidology. (1977). *Suicide and how to prevent it*. West Point, PA: Merck, Sharp, and Dome.

American Association of Suicidology (AAS) Public Information Committee. (1987). Preliminary guidelines for media developed. *Newslink, 13*(2), 10.

American Psychiatric Association. (1987). *Diagnostic and statistical manual of mental disorders* (3rd ed., rev.). Washington, DC: Author.

Baron, C. (1986). Child welfare league conference looks at teen suicide. *The Network News, 3*, 4–5.

Barrett, T. (1985a). Does suicide prevention in the schools have to be a "terrifying" concept? *Newslink, 11*(1), 3.

Barrett, T. (1985b). *Youth in crisis: Seeking solutions to self-destructive behavior*. Longmont, CO: Sopris West.

Beck, A., Schuyler, R., & Herman, J. (1974). Development of suicidal intent scales. In A. Beck, H. Resnick, & D. Lettieri (Eds.), *The prediction of suicide*. Springfield, IL: Charles C. Thomas.

Berkovitz, I. (1985). The role of the schools in child, adolescent and youth suicide prevention. In M. Peck, N. Farberow, & R. Litman (Eds.), *Youth suicide* (pp. 170–181). New York: Springer.

Berman, L. (1985). Youth suicide: On hyperbole and public miseducation. *Newslink, 11*(4), 3.

Berman, L. (1986). AAS plans model school suicide program. *Newslink, 12*(4), 1.

Berman, L. (1987a, Fall). Adolescent suicide: Clinical consultation. *The Clinical Psychologist*, pp. 87–89.

Berman, L. (1987b, November). Suicide prevention: A critical need and a critical perspective. In A. McEvoy (Chair), *Suicide prevention and the schools*. Symposium sponsored by Learning Publications, Orlando, FL.

Biblarz, D. (1988, April). Not in my school: Entry issues. In S. Perlin (Chair), *Tackling the tough issues in school based suicide awareness programs*. Symposium conducted at the meeting of the American Association of Suicidology, Washington, DC.

Bishop, J. (1986, September 11). Rise in suicide by teenagers is noted in wake of TV programs on the subject. *The Wall Street Journal*, p. 14.

Boggs, M. (1987). *Suicide prevention in educational settings.* Unpublished manuscript, Suicide Prevention Center, Dayton, OH.

Bolton, I. (1987). Beyond surviving: Suggestions for survivors. In J. Dunne, J. McIntosh, & K. Dunne-Maxim (Eds.), *Suicide and its aftermath* (pp. 289–290). New York: Norton.

Bonner, R. L. (1987). Everyone knows asking people about thoughts of suicide won't put the idea in their heads—don't they? *Newslink, 13*(2), 8–12.

Boyd, J., & Mościcki, E. (1986). Firearms and youth suicide. *American Journal of Public Health, 76,* 1240–1242.

Brown, S. (1987). Sample interview questions for assessing suicidal risk. *The Network News, 6,* 5–6.

Brown, S., & Schroff, B. (1986). Taking care of ourselves. *The Network News, 4,* 5–6.

California State Department of Education. (1987). *Suicide prevention program for the California public schools.* Sacramento: Author.

Cantor, P. (1985, February 18). These teenagers feel they have no options. *People,* pp. 84–87.

Cantor, P. (1987, November). Communication with students at risk. In A. McEvoy (Chair), *Suicide prevention and the schools.* Symposium sponsored by Learning Publications, Orlando, FL.

Caplan, G. (1964). *Principles of preventive psychiatry.* New York: Basic Books.

Capuzzi, D. (1987, November). Intervention strategies for youth at risk. In A. McEvoy (Chair), *Suicide prevention and the schools.* Symposium sponsored by Learning Publications, Orlando, FL.

Centers for Disease Control (CDC). (1986). *Youth suicide in the United States, 1970 to 1980.* Atlanta: Author.

Chambers, W., Purg-Antich, J., & Tabrizi, M. (1978). *The ongoing development of the kiddie-SADS.* Paper presented at the annual meeting of the American Academy of Child Psychiatry, San Diego.

Childress, J. (1985). Ethical issues. In N. Farberow, S. Altman, & A. Thorne (Eds.), *Report of the National Conference on Youth Suicide* (pp. 303–309). Washington, DC: Youth Suicide National Center.

Cohen, D., & Poland, S. (1988). [Suicide survey results]. Unpublished raw data.

Coleman, L. (1987a). Beyond Bergenfield: Making sense of suicide clusters. *The Network News, 7,* 1–5.

Coleman, L. (1987b). *Suicide clusters.* Boston: Faber & Faber.

Colt, G. (1984). Youth: What quality pain? *Newslink, 10*(4), 1–3.

Colt, H. (1986). The enigma of suicide. In J. Fencik (Ed.), *A teachers' manual for the prevention of suicide among adolescents* (pp. 31–63). Providence, RI: Samaritans.

Comstock, B. (1985). Youth suicide cluster: A community response. *Newslink, 2*(2), 6.

Coronet Films (Producer). (1984). *Suicide—the warning signs* [Film]. Northbrook, IL: Producer.

Crabb, A. (1982, February). Children and environmental disasters: The counselor's responsibility. *Elementary School Guidance and Counseling,* pp. 228–231.

Cull, J., & Gill, W. (1982). *Suicide probability scale manual.* Los Angeles: Western Publishing Services.

Davidson, H. (1985). Legal issues. In N. Farberow, S. Altman, & A. Thorne (Eds.), *Report of the National Conference on Youth Suicide* (pp. 297–303). Washington, DC: Youth Suicide National Center.

Davis, J. (1985). Suicidal crises in schools. *School Psychology Review, 14,* 313–324.

Davis, J., Sandoval, J., & Wilson, M. (1988). Strategies for the primary prevention of adolescent suicide. *School Psychology Review, 17,* 559–569.

Denver Post. (1987, March 27). "Teacher put on leave after her pupil's suicide," p. 6a.

Doyle, N. (1987). *Confidentiality.* Unpublished manuscript, Huntington School District, Huntington, NY.

Dunne-Maxim, K. (1985). The New Jersey plan. In N. Farberow, S. Altman, & A. Thorne (Eds.), *Report of the National Conference on Youth Suicide* (pp. 183–187). Washington, DC: Youth Suicide National Center.

Dunne-Maxim, K. (1987, November). Postvention in the schools. In A. McEvoy (Chair), *Suicide prevention and the schools.* Symposium sponsored by Learning Publications, Orlando, FL.

Dunne-Maxim, K., Dunne, E., & Hauser, M. (1987). When children are survivors. In E. Dunne, J. McIntosh, & K. Dunne-Maxim (Eds.), *Suicide and its aftermath* (pp. 234–245). New York: Norton.

Elkind, D. (1978). *The child's reality: Three developmental themes.* New York: Wiley.

Engelman, R. (1987). Running away from home is a sign of suicidal bent. *The Network News, 7,* 9.

Eyeman, J. (1987, March). Pre-conference workshop. *Suicide prevention in schools.* Symposium presented at the meeting of the National Association of School Psychologists, New Orleans.

Fairfax County Public Schools. (1987). *The adolescent suicide prevention program.* Fairfax, VA: Author.

Farberow, N., Altman, S., & Thorne, A. (Eds.). (1985). *Report of the National Conference on Youth Suicide.* Washington, DC: Youth Suicide National Center.

Felner, R. (1987, November). Primary prevention of youth suicide. In A. McEvoy (Chair), *Suicide prevention and the schools.* Symposium sponsored by Learning Publications, Orlando, FL.

Fencik, J. (Ed.). (1986). *A teacher's manual for the prevention of suicide among adolescents.* Providence, RI: Samaritans.

Fortinsky, R. (1987). U.S.M. study finds link between runaways and suicidal potential. *The Network News, 7,* 9.

Friedman, R., Corn, R., Jurt, S., Fibel, B., Schulick, J., & Swirsky, S. (1984). Family history of illness in the seriously suicidal adolescent: A life-cycle approach. *American Journal of Orthopsychiatry, 54,* 390–397.

Friend, T. (1988, December 5). *More teens are dying violently. USA Today,* p. 1d.

Garfinkel, B. (1986, June). *School based prevention programs.* Paper presented at the National Conference on Prevention and Intervention in Youth Suicide, Oakland, CA.

Garland, A. (1987, November). Prevention programs: Evaluation guidelines. In A. McEvoy (Chair), *Suicide prevention and the schools.* Symposium sponsored by Learning Publications, Orlando, FL.

Giffin, M., & Felsenthal, C. (1983). *A cry for help.* New York: Doubleday.

Gordon, S. (1985). *When living hurts.* New York: Union of Hebrew Congregations.

Gould, M., & Shaffer, D. (1986). The impact of suicide in television movies: Evidence of imitation. *New England Journal of Medicine, 315,* 690–694.

Guetzloe, E. (1988). Suicide and depression: Special education's responsibility. *Teaching Exceptional Children, 20*(4), 24–29.

Guetzloe, E. (in press). *Youth suicide: What the educator should know.* Reston, VA: Council for Exceptional Children.

Gumbleton, G., & Elchinger, H. (1987). Anatomy of a crisis. *California Association of School Psychology Today, 37*(1), 24–26.

Hardy, M. (1985). Students Against Suicide. In N. Farberow, S. Altman, & A. Thorne (Eds.), *Report of the National Conference on Youth Suicide* (pp. 279–283). Washington, DC: Youth Suicide National Center.

Harkavy-Friedman, J., Asnis, G., Boek, M., & DiFiore, J. (1987). Prevalence of specific suicidal behaviors in a high school sample. *American Journal of Psychiatry, 144,* 1203–1206.

Harnisch, P. (1987). Conference highlights AAS/IAS. *Newslink, 13*(2), 1–2.

Harris, M., & Crawford, R. (1987). *Youth suicide: The identification of effective concepts and practices in policies and procedures for Texas schools* (Monograph No. 3). Commerce: Center for Policy Studies and Research, East Texas State University.

Heckler, M. (1985). A greeting to the conference. In N. Farberow, S. Altman, & A. Thorne (Eds.), *Report of the National Conference on Youth Suicide* (pp. xxxi–xxxiv). Washington, DC: Youth Suicide National Center.

Helman, M., Jones, F., Lamb, F., Dunne-Maxim, K., & Sutton, C. (1985). A training model for school personnel. In N. Farberow, S. Altman, & A. Thorne (Eds.), *Report of the National Conference on Youth Suicide* (pp. 265–274). Washington, DC: Youth Suicide National Center.

Hellmich, N. (1988, August 10). One in seven teens say they've tried suicide. *USA Today,* p. 1.

Hidlay, W. (1988, September 14). Even the brightest teens consider suicide, poll says. *Houston Chronicle,* p. 1d.

Hendin, H. (1987). Youth suicide: A psychosocial perspective. *Suicide and Life-Threatening Behavior, 17,* 151–166.

Henegar, C. (1986). Suicides in the shelters: Liability in the runaway centers. *The Network News, 4,* 4–7.

Hill, W. (1984). Intervention and postvention in schools. In H. Sudak, A. Ford, & N. Rushforth (Eds.), *Suicide in the young* (pp. 407–416). Boston: John Wright.

Hipple, J. (1983, Fall). Counseling suicidal individuals. *Texas Professional Guidance Association Journal,* pp. 93–102.

Hipple, J., & Cimbolic, P. (1979). *The counselor and suicidal crisis.* Springfield, IL: Charles C Thomas.

Hoff, L. (1978). *People in crisis: Understanding and helping.* Reading, MA: Addison-Wesley.

Houston Post. (1988, March 5). "13-year-old girl commits suicide after classmates find her diary," p. 9a.

Houston Post. (1987, September 21). "Ex-husband sued over suicide," p. 11a.

Houston Post. (1988, January 22). "Mother sentenced to year in prison over teen's suicide," p. 13a.

Indiana State Board of Health. (Ed.). (1985). *A school approach for the prevention of youth suicide.* Unpublished manuscript.

Inwald, R., Brobst, K., & Morrissey, R. (1987). *Hilson adolescent profile manual.* Kew Gardens, NJ: Hilson Research, Inc.

Jackson, V. (1988). [Interview with the author about a school crisis in Katy, TX.]

Jacobs, J. (1971). *Adolescent suicide.* New York: Wiley.

Johnson, D. (1987, February 8). Student's suicide leads to lawsuit. *New York Times*, p. 3a.

Johnson, S., & Maile, L. (1987). *Suicide and the schools.* Springfield, IL: Charles C Thomas.

Kahn, A. (1985). The role of the PTA and youth suicide prevention. In N. Farberow, S. Altman, & A. Thorne (Eds.), *Report of the National Conference on Youth Suicide* (pp. 197–200). Washington, DC: Youth Suicide National Center.

Klagsburn, F. (1976). *Too young to die: Youth and suicide.* Boston: Houghton Mifflin.

Kniesel, D., & Richards, G. (1988). Crisis intervention after the suicide of a teacher. *Professional Psychology: Research and Practice, 19*(2), 165–169.

Kubler-Ross, E. (1969). *On death and dying.* New York: Macmillan.

Lamartine, C. (1985). Suicide prevention in educational settings. In *After a suicide death* (pamphlet). Dayton, OH: Suicide Prevention Center.

Lamb, F., & Dunne-Maxim, K. (1987). Postvention in the schools: Policy and process. In E. Dunne, J. McIntosh, & K. Dunne-Maxim (Eds.), *Suicide and its aftermath* (pp. 245–263). New York: Norton.

Landis, L. (1987a). House conducts teen suicide hearings. *Guideposts, 29*(18), 3.

Landis, L. (1987b). Suicide epidemic spreading among nation's teenagers. *Guideposts, 30*(3), 16.

Leahy, T. (1985). Media: Corporate concern. In N. Farberow, S. Altman, & A. Thorne (Eds.), *Report of the National Conference on Youth Suicide* (pp. 229–235). Washington, DC: Youth Suicide National Center.

Leder, M. (1987). *Dead serious: A book for teenagers about teenage suicide.* New York: Atheneum.

Lennox, C. (1987). *Guidelines for high school suicide prevention programs.* Unpublished doctoral dissertation, East Texas State University.

Lester, D. (1988). Research note: Gun control, gun ownership and suicide prevention. *Suicide and Life-Threatening Behavior, 18*, 176–181.

Lindborg, S., & Wagner, N. (1987). *Suicide prevention and intervention* (Monograph No. 2). Minneapolis: Minnesota School Psychology Association.

Lindegard, J. (1986). Who's Who among American High School Student's (20th ed.). Lake Forest, IL: Educational Communications, Inc.

Lindeman, E., & Greer, I. (1972). A study of grief: Emotional responses to suicide. In A. Cain (Ed.), *Survivors of suicide* (pp. 63–69). Springfield, IL: Charles C Thomas.

Lipton, T., & Leader, E. (1985). Teen Line: A mental health delivery system for youth. In N. Farberow, S. Altman, & A. Thorne (Eds.), *Report of the National Conference on Youth Suicide* (pp. 219–223). Washington, DC: Youth Suicide National Center.

Livingston, D. (1985). Foreword. In N. Farberow, S. Altman, & A. Thorne (Eds.), *Report of the National Conference on Youth Suicide* (pp. xix–xx). Washington, DC: Youth Suicide National Center.

Looney, J., Oldham, D., Claman, L., Crumley, F., & Waller, D. (1985). Suicide by adolescents. *Texas Medicine, 81,* 45–49.

Maris, R. (1985). The adolescent suicide problem. *Suicide and Life-Threatening Behavior, 15,* 91–109.

McBrien, J. (1983). Are you thinking of killing yourself?: Confronting students' suicidal thoughts. *The School Counselor, 31*(1), 79–82.

McDermott, J. (1987). Fantasy game may promote cognitive skill in many young people. *Clinical Psychiatry News, 14*(12), 635–647.

McGinnis, J. (1987). Suicide in America—moving up the public health agenda. *Suicide and Life-Threatening Behavior, 17,* 18–32.

McKinney, G. (1985). Florida state plan. In N. Farberow, S. Altman, & A. Thorne (Eds.), *Report of the National Conference on Youth Suicide* (pp. 179–183). Washington, DC: Youth Suicide National Center.

Mulholland, R. (1986, September 19). We must face suicide, not hide it. *USA Today,* p. 10a.

National Coalition on Television Violence. (1987, May 12). Dungeons and dragons fantasy role-playing linked to 90 deaths: Groups plead for hearings (press release). Champaign, IL.

National Committee on Youth Suicide Prevention and American Association of Suicidology (Producers). (1987). *Young people in crisis* [Film]. Staten Island, NY: Exar Communications.

National Center for Health Statistics. (1980). [Nationwide Suicide Statistics (ages 10–24)]. Unpublished raw data.

National Institute of Mental Health. (1985). *Suicide in the United States: 1958–1982.* Washington, DC: Government Printing Office.

Nelson, F., Faberow, N., & Litman, R. (1987). Youth suicide in California. In R. Yufit (Ed.), *Proceedings of the Twentieth Annual Conference of the American Association of Suicidology* (pp. 296–297). San Francisco: American Association of Suicidology.

O'Connor, M. (1985). The California model. In N. Farberow, S. Altman, & A. Thorne (Eds.), *Report of the National Conference on Youth Suicide* (pp. 173–179). Washington, DC: Youth Suicide National Center.

O'Dell (1985, January 6). Bright, popular Ozark student falls to dark, lonely thoughts. Springfield (Missouri) *News-Leader*, p. 1.

Office of the Inspector General (OIG). (1986). *Youth suicide: National program inspection*. Seattle: Author.

Orbach, I., & Glaubman, H. (1979). The concept of death and suicidal behavior in young children. *Journal of the American Academy of Child Psychiatry, 18*, 668–678.

Painter, K. (1987, September 24). Teen suicide isn't triggered by TV movies. *USA Today*, p. 1a.

Peck, M. (1985). California Youth Suicide Prevention Program. In N. Farberow, S. Altman, & A. Thorne (Eds.), *Report of the National Conference on Youth Suicide* (pp. 261–265). Washington, DC: Youth Suicide National Center.

Peck, M., Farberow, N., & Litman, R. (Eds.). (1985). *Youth suicide*. New York: Springer.

Pelej, J., & Scholzen, K. (1987). Postvention: A schools response to suicide. In R. Yufit (Ed.), *Proceedings of the Twentieth Annual Conference of the American Association of Suicidology* (pp. 387–390). San Francisco: American Association of Suicidology.

Perlman, J. (1987). Golden Gate Bridge: Site of beauty and despair. *Newslink, 13*(11).

Pfeffer, C. (1986). *The suicidal child*. New York: Guilford Press.

Phillips, B. (1988). [Interview with author about media coverage of a suicide in Austin, TX.]

Phillips, D. (1986, September 19). Media attention helps encourage teen suicide. *USA Today*, p. 10a.

Phillips, D., & Carstensen, L. (1986). Clustering of teenage suicides after television news stories about suicide. *New England Journal of Medicine, 315*, 685–689.

Phillips, D., & Carstensen, L. (1988). The effect of suicide stories on various demographic groups, 1968–1985. *Suicide and Life-Threatening Behavior, 18*, 100–112.

Phillips, D., & Willis, J. (1987). A drop in suicides around major national holidays. *Suicide and Life-Threatening Behavior, 17*, 1–13.

Porter, W. (1985). *Inservice and resource guide for children and adolescent suicide prevention*. Unpublished manuscript, Cherry Creek Schools, Denver, CO.

Radecki, T. (1986). *Deer Hunter* deaths climb to 43. *National Coalition on Television Violence News, 7*(1), 2.

Reynolds, W. (1987). *Suicidal ideation questionnaire*. Odessa, FL: Psychological Assessment Resources, Inc.

Richman, J. (1986). *Family and therapy for suicidal people*. New York: Springer.

Ring, J. (1985). Working with the media. In Indiana State Board of Health (Ed.), *A school approach for the prevention of youth suicide*. Unpublished manuscript.

Ross, C. (1985a). Teaching children the facts of life and death: Suicide prevention in the schools. In M. Peck, N. Farberow, & R. Litman (Eds.), *Youth suicide* (pp. 147–169). New York: Springer.

Ross, C. (1985b). The Youth Suicide National Center. In N. Farberow, S. Altman, & A. Thorne (Eds.), *Report of the National Conference on Youth Suicide* (pp. 315–321). Washington, DC: Youth Suicide National Center.

Ross, C. (1985c). Foreword. In N. Farberow, S. Altman, & A. Thorne (Eds.), *Report of the National Conference on Youth Suicide* (pp. xxi–xxvii). Washington, DC: Youth Suicide National Center.

Ruof, S., & Harris, J. (1988a). Questions and answers on legal issues related to suicide. *Communique, 16*(6), 18.

Ruof, S., & Harris, J. (1988b). Suicide contagion: Guilt and modeling. *Communique, 16*(17), 8.

Ruof, S., Harris, J., & Robbie, M. (1987). *Handbook: Suicide prevention in the school*. LaSalle, CO: Weld Boces.

Ryerson, D. (1987, November). Schools and community based organizations working toward suicide prevention. In A. McEvoy (Chair), *Suicide prevention and the schools*. Symposium sponsored by Learning Publications, Orlando, FL.

Ryerson, D. (1988, April). The importance of school personnel and researchers collaborating. In K. Smith (Chair), *How do we know what we've done? Controversy in evaluation*. Symposium conducted at the Meeting of the American Association of Suicidology, Washington, DC.

Schafly, P. (1985). The school and youth suicide. In N. Farberow, S. Altman, & A. Thorne (Eds.), *Report of the National Conference on Youth Suicide* (pp. 269–275). Washington, DC: Youth Suicide National Center.

Schindler, R., & Poland, S. (1985). *Teenage suicide prevention tips*. Unpublished manuscript, Cypress–Fairbanks Independent School District, Cypress, TX.

Schutz, B. (1982). *Legal liability in psychotherapy*. San Francisco: Jossey-Bass.

Scobie, W. (1986). California case becomes focus of concern over youth suicide. *The Network News, 3*, 12–13.

Seibel, M., & Murray, J. (1988, March). Early prevention of adolescent suicide. *Educational Leadership*, pp. 48–51.

Shaffer, D. (1988, April). School research issues. In K. Smith (Chair), *How do we know what we've done? Controversy in evaluation*. Symposium conducted at the Meeting of the American Association of Suicidology, Washington, DC.

Sharlin, S., & Shenhar, A. (1986). The fusion of pressing situation and releasing writing: On adolescent suicide poetry. *Suicide and Life-Threatening Behavior, 16*, 343–355.

Shipman, F. (1987). Student stress and suicide. *The Practitioner, 14*(2), 1–10.

Shneidman, E. (1985). *Definition of suicide*. New York: Wiley.

Slenkovitch, J. (1986, June). School districts can be sued for inadequate suicide prevention programs. *The Schools' Advocate*, pp. 1–3.

Small, A. H., & Small, A. D. (1984). Children's reactions to a suicide in the family and the implications for treatment. In N. Linzer (Ed.), *Suicide: The will to live vs. the will to die* (pp. 151–169). New York: Human Sciences Press.

Smith, J. (1987). [Interview with author about Dallas, TX, School Prevention Program].

Smith, J. (1988a). *Suicide risk assessment worksheet.* Unpublished manuscript, Dallas Independent School District, Dallas, TX.

Smith, J. (1988b). *A crisis intervention curriculum for teenagers and young adults.* Holmes Beach, FL: Learning Publications Inc.

Smith, K. (1985, November). *Child suicide: Issues in assessment and treatment.* Paper presented at Child Suicide: A conference of Hope, Houston.

Smith, K. (Chair). (1988, April). *How do we know what we've done? Controversy in evaluation.* Symposium conducted at the meeting of the American Association of Suicidology, Washington, DC.

Smith, K., & Crawford, S. (1986). Suicidal behavior among "normal" high school students. *Suicide and Life-Threatening Behavior, 16,* 313–325.

Smith, K., Eyeman, J., Dyck, R., & Ryerson, D. (1987). *Report of the School Suicide Programs Questionnaire.* Unpublished manuscript.

South Bergen Mental Health Center (1987). *Adolescent suicide prevention program for school communities.* Lyndhurst, NJ: South Bergen.

Sowers, J. (1987, November). Issues in curriculum and program development. In A. McEvoy (Chair), *Suicide prevention and the schools.* Symposium sponsored by Learning Publications, Orlando, FL.

Sowers, J. (1988, April). What is needed in the curriculum. In J. Kalafat (Chair), *Who, what, and how: Curriculum development and program content.* Symposium conducted at the meeting of the American Association of Suicidology, Washington, DC.

Spitzzeri, A. (1987). Psychologist suspended for failure to disclose confidential information. *Communique, 16*(2), 5–6.

Spoonhour, A. (1985, February 18). Teen suicide. *People,* pp. 76–83.

Stanton, J., & Stanton, S. (1987). Family and system therapy of suicidal adolescents. *Family Therapy Today, 2*(11), 1–4.

Stark, K. (Chair). (1987, May). *Depression and children.* Symposium presented at the meeting of the Texas Psychology Association, School Psychology Division, Houston.

Suicide essay ends tragically: Boy describes own death. (1986, March 21). *Houston Post,* p. 8a.

Sunburst Communications (Producer). (1985). *Teens who choose life* [Film]. Pleasantville, NY: Producer.

Tanney, B. (1988, April). School curriculum approaches. In J. Kalafat (Chair), *Who, what, and how: Curriculum development and program content.* Symposium conducted at the meeting of the American Association of Suicidology, Washington, DC.

Toolan, J. (1975). Suicide in children and adolescents. *American Journal of Psychotherapy, 29,* 339–344.

Tugend, A. (1984). Schools, mental health experts grappling with the last taboo. *Education Week, 4*(9), 1–13.

Underwood, M., Jakubik, C., & Kalafat, J. (1985). *Lifelines: Sequential curricula on adolescent suicide.* Denville, NJ: St. Clare's Hospital.

U.S.A. Today. (1987, August 21). "Lost years to suicide," p. 1a.

U.S.A. Today. (1987, April 21). "Suicidal thoughts of our teenagers," p. 1a.

Vidal, J. (1986, October). Establishing a suicide prevention program. *National Association of Secondary School Principals Bulletin,* pp. 68–72.

Withers, L., & Kaplan, D. (1987). Adolescents who attempt suicide: A retrospective clinical chart review of hospitalized patients. *Professional Psychology: Research and Practice, 18,* 391–393.

Wisconsin Department of Instruction. (1986). *Suicide prevention: A resource and planning guide.* Madison: Author.

Worden, J. (1982). *Grief counseling and grief therapy.* New York: Springer.

World Health Organization. (1977). *International classification of diseases* (9th ed.). Geneva: Author.

Index

19.95